W9-BUY-119

PRAISE FOR INTEGRAL HEALTH

*"This is a wise and gentle book of healing,
grounded in experience, rich with practice,
deeply hopeful. Read it. Savor it. Share it."*

—JAMES S. GORDON, M.D.
FOUNDER AND DIRECTOR, CENTER FOR MIND-BODY MEDICINE
AUTHOR OF *MANIFESTO FOR A NEW MEDICINE*
FORMER CHAIR WHITE HOUSE COMMISSION ON COMPLEMENTARY
AND ALTERNATIVE MEDICINE POLICY

*"Dr. Elliott Dacher has written a book that is more than a truly
brilliant guide to mind-body balance and healing. It's rich
with humanity, a testimony to the wisdom and compassion
of this extraordinary physician and spiritual teacher."*

—JOAN BORYSENKO, PH.D.
AUTHOR OF *MINDING THE BODY, MENDING THE MIND* AND
INNER PEACE FOR BUSY PEOPLE

*"Integral Health is a precious gift from a master healer written
in the voice of a soulful poet and dedicated teacher. Dacher calls
us to a transformation in self and society that can promote nothing
less than human flourishing. There is something here that speaks
to anyone who has ever wondered what medicine might
become if it promoted the fullness of our being."*

—MARILYN SCHLITZ, PH.D.
VICE-PRESIDENT FOR RESEARCH AND EDUCATION INSTITUTE OF NOETIC SCIENCES
AUTHOR OF *CONSCIOUSNESS AND HEALING*

*"Integral Health is a soaring, lyrical journey that will
awaken you to the job of being alive. It will also help
you become a wiser, healthier person who is attuned
to what really matters. Highly recommended."*

—BARBARA DOSSEY, PH.D., R.N.
DIRECTOR, HOLISTIC NURSING CONSULTANTS
AUTHOR OF *HOLISTIC NURSING: A HANDBOOK FOR PRACTICE*
AND *FLORENCE NIGHTINGALE: MYSTIC, VISIONARY, HEALER*

"This book provides the operating system for integral medicine and for transforming both medicine and ourselves as healers. Dr. Dacher's deep knowledge of personal transformational practices, of diverse healing systems, and of philosopher Ken Wilber's integral model join hands in a book of marvelous significance that will help change our world for the better. Thank you, Elliott, for the work you do."

VICTOR S. SIERPINA, M.D.
W.D. AND LAURA NELL NICHOLSON FAMILY PROFESSOR OF INTEGRATIVE MEDICINE
UNIVERSITY OF TEXAS MEDICAL BRANCH, GALVESTON, TEXAS

"Dr. Dacher has clearly written another eye-opening book as he tackles old 20th-century assumptions about what constitutes good health and full human potential. . . ."

MARC S. MICOZZI, M.D., PH.D.
AUTHOR OF *FUNDAMENTALS OF COMPLEMENTARY AND INTEGRATIVE MEDICINE,* 3RD EDITION

"We are living in a remarkable time of increasing medical miracles but diminishing patient satisfaction. Finally, one of our own has come to the rescue with wisdom and sensitivity. In his new book Integral Health, Dacher has given us direction for the future so that we might once again come alive to all the needs of our patients and understand the spiritual connections that are the root cause of many modern illnesses. This is a book for both patients and healers. It should be required reading for medical administrators, insurers, and healthcare policy makers."

—STEVEN F. HOROWITZ, M.D.
CLINICAL PROFESSOR OF MEDICINE, ALBERT EINSTEIN COLLEGE OF MEDICINE
CHIEF OF CARDIOLOGY AT THE STAMFORD HOSPITAL, STAMFORD, CONNECTICUT

"Dr. Elliott Dacher is an experienced and soulful American physician who has immersed himself in the spiritual traditions of the world, most recently spending long periods of time in the East with his spiritual community. Dr. Dacher comes back to us with a simple yet profound message—that our lives are precious, and if we embrace that fully, we can direct our lives toward better health, deeper love, and greater joy. A deeply moving and healing book for all, I highly recommend it."

—MARTIN L. ROSSMAN, M.D.
UCSF MEDICAL SCHOOL, AUTHOR OF *GUIDED IMAGERY FOR SELF-HEALING*
AND *FIGHTING CANCER FROM WITHIN*

INTEGRAL HEALTH

The Path to Human Flourishing

ELLIOTT S. DACHER, M.D.

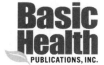

Basic Health
PUBLICATIONS, INC.

The information contained in this book is based upon the research and personal and professional experiences of the author. It is not intended as a substitute for consulting with your physician or other healthcare provider. Any attempt to diagnose and treat an illness should be done under the direction of a healthcare professional.

The publisher does not advocate the use of any particular healthcare protocol but believes the information in this book should be available to the public. The publisher and author are not responsible for any adverse effects or consequences resulting from the use of the suggestions, preparations, or procedures discussed in this book. Should the reader have any questions concerning the appropriateness of any procedures or preparation mentioned, the author and the publisher strongly suggest consulting a professional healthcare advisor.

Material on page 29 from Edelstein, Emma J., and Ludwig Edelstein. *Asclepius: Collection and Interpretation of the Testimonies,* pp. 212. © 1998 [Copyright Holder] Reprinted with permission of the Johns Hopkins University Press.

Material on page 89 from *The Selected Poetry of Rainer Maria Rilke* by Rainer Maria Rilke, translated by Stephen Mitchel, copyright © 1982 by Stephen Mitchel. Used by permission of Random House, Inc.

Material on page 102 from *Letters to a Young Poet* by Rainer Maria Rilke, translated by M.D. Herter Norton. Copyright © 1934, 1954 by W.W. Norton & Company, Inc., renewed © 1962, 1982 by M.D. Herter Norton. Used by permission of W.W. Norton, Inc.

Material on pages 102 and 103 from *The Prophet* by Kahlil Gibran, copyright © 1923 by Kahlil Gibran 1923 and renewed by Administrators C.T.A. of Kahlil Gibran Estate and Mary G. Gibran. Used by permission of Alfred A Knopf, a division of Random House, Inc.

Material on page 157 from *A Sleep of Prisoners* by Christopher Fry, Copyright © renewed 1979, 1989, Christopher Fry. Copyright © 1951, 1953 Christopher Fry.

Material on page 158 from *Integral Healing, Sri Aurobindo and the Mother,* page 227. Published by Sri Aurobindo Ashram Publication Department, Pondicherry, India, 2004. Used by permission from Sri Aurobindo Ashram Trust.

Basic Health Publications, Inc.

28812 Top of the World Drive • Laguna Beach, CA 92651 • 949-715-7327

Library of Congress Cataloging-in-Publication Data

Dacher, Elliott S.
    Integral health : the path to human flourishing / Elliott S. Dacher.
        p. cm.
    Includes bibliographical references and index.
    ISBN-13: 978-1-59120-190-8
    ISBN-10: 1-59120-190-X
    1. Health—Philosophy. 2. Consciousness. 3. Holistic medicine.
4. Alternative medicine. I. Title.

    RA776.5.D334   2006
    610—dc22

                                        2006007485

Copyright © 2006 by Elliott S. Dacher, M.D.

All rights reserved. No part of this publication may be reproduced, stored in a retrieval system, or transmitted, in any form or by any means, electronic, mechanical, photocopying, recording, or otherwise, without the prior written consent of the copyright owner.

Editor: Susan Davis • Copyeditor: Carol Rosenberg
Interior graphics: Jessica Dacher (www.design.jumbojessie.com)
Typesetting/Book design: Gary A. Rosenberg • Cover design: Mike Stromberg

Printed in the United States of America

10   9   8   7   6   5   4   3   2   1

Contents

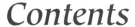
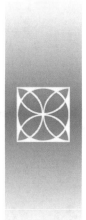

A Letter to the Reader, 1

The Vision

Chapter 1:   This Precious Life, 7

Chapter 2:   Consciousness and Health, 15

Chapter 3:   Aesclepian Healing, 25

The Path

Chapter 4:   Integral Healing, 35

Chapter 5:   Preparing the Ground, 49

Chapter 6:   Psychospiritual Flourishing, 59

Chapter 7:   The Subtle Mind, 71

Chapter 8:   Biological Flourishing, 79

Chapter 9:   Interpersonal Flourishing, 87

Chapter 10:   Flourishing in the World, 95

Chapter 11:   The Integral Assessment, 105

Chapter 12:   Integral Practice, 117

Chapter 13:   The Four Essential Points, 129

The Fruits

Chapter 14:   Human Flourishing, 139

Chapter 15:   The Center for Human Flourishing, 147

Chapter 16:   Life Divine, 155

Appendices

Appendix A: The Evolution of Medicine, 159

Appendix B: For the Practitioner, 165

Resource Guide, 175

Acknowledgments, 179

Index, 181

About the Author, 184

And so I join my hands and pray . . .
For all those ailing in the world,
Until their every sickness has been healed,
May I myself become for them
The doctor, the nurse, the medicine itself.

—SHANTIDEVA

A Letter to
the Reader

Dear Reader:

I invite you to join me on a journey of self-transformation. We begin this journey with a simple yet profound acknowledgment—all of us want a life of authentic health, happiness, and wholeness. We want to go beyond our usual sense of health and life. We want to live with purpose, passion, intimacy, and joy.

But you have to want that with your whole being. You have to want that more than the comfort of what you now know because authentic health will change you. Conventional health is simple. Just follow what you've learned. A far-reaching health requires a transformation of mind and heart. We call this holistic and evolutionary transformation an integral shift. The result is integral health. This deep challenge can open new realms of health and healing. It requires that we be open, receptive, daring, and bold.

What is holding us back? Why have we settled for ordinary health when so much more is possible? The answer is so close that it is difficult for us to see. We've been trained to deal with suffering, distress, and disease by looking outside of ourselves by relying on remedies, therapies, techniques, health practitioners, self-help, and self-improvement programs. We've been similarly trained to look outward for "happiness," seeking pleasure from materialism, success, fame, romance, sexuality, alcohol, and drugs. But temporary relief and ephemeral pleasures that can comfort us for moments cannot transform ordinary health into enduring, exceptional health.

For this we need to redirect our efforts. We've been looking *outward* toward worldly experiences rather than *inward* toward our essence. That is our dilemma in the West. We have gained mastery over the physical and lost touch with the spiritual. *To transform health and life we must shift our gaze inward, where we will find the ever-present source of exceptional health and healing.*

Consider the journey of this well-intentioned internist from outer healing to inner healing to whole healing. I practiced internal medicine from 1975 to 1996. During this period, I participated in more than 45,000 office visits. From the very beginning, I came face-to-face with the enormous complexity of mental distress and physical disease that my medical education sanitized and reduced to a simple, yet incomplete biological diagnosis and requisite therapy.

Before long, it became apparent that I had been inadequately prepared to care for others' lives—both their presenting symptoms and their larger possibilities. I saw this played out in my office each day. It was the patient with a stomach ulcer whose ulcerated life went unseen; the middle-aged man with heart disease whose heart, broken by years of meaningless toil, went uncared for; and the man or woman who did not fit into a neat diagnostic category yet was nevertheless suffering from disabling fatigue, pervasive anxiety, or unrelenting low-level depression.

They wanted what we all want—health, happiness, and wholeness. I would catch a glimpse of this longing in a facial expression, in the way the body was held, and in a silent reaching out. In my consulting room, this yearning of soul and spirit was translated into physical symptoms and then reduced by custom to a diagnostic label. The deeper source of these ailments went unseen, unheard, and overlooked. In time, I came to recognize that I did not understand or even have the tools with which to address this deeper yearning.

As a result of these experiences, I began a journey of discovery. I read as much as I could about stress, an obvious underlying issue in most of my patients. This interest extended to the study of developmental psychology, wellness, mind/body healing, and then finally consciousness and health. I slowly incorporated some of these understandings and practices into my work with patients and authored two books, *Intentional Healing* and *Whole Healing*. I spoke extensively throughout the country on these new approaches. I thought I finally understood the deeper and more profound aspects of health and healing, but I was wrong. There was still a distance to go, yet another education—one that reached further inside.

Ten years ago, I began what I consider to be my second medical education, this time in the East. The Eastern philosophies spoke to me about wisdom, compassion, the alleviation of needless suffering, and the promotion of sustained health, happiness, and wholeness. This second medical education focused on the inner rather than the outer, the mind rather than the body. Its goal was the permanent alleviation of unnecessary suffering and the promotion of human flourishing.

I made many trips abroad to study the philosophy of human flourishing. It was there that I saw firsthand the living reality of exceptional health and well-being. This flourishing of body, mind, and spirit was self-cultivated rather than reliant on outer remedies, permanent rather than transitory, hardy rather than fragile, and capable of surfing rather than succumbing to life's adversities—including disease, aging, and death. This discovery and the gradual familiarity with its methods and practices were the focus of my second medical education.

I now know with certainty that humanity's yearning for profound health and life can be realized in our lifetime. With access to the West's mastery of outer science *and* the East's mastery of inner science, we *can* evolve to the next level of health.

In the following pages, we will explore the vision and practices that enable us to take this important path toward integral health. Together we will begin this last leg of humankind's long journey from survival to modern diagnostics to human flourishing.

How do we take this noble vision of exceptional health and translate it into a practical possibility? For this we need a map. The map that we use is based on Ken Wilber's integral theory. It is a comprehensive and far-reaching approach to health and healing that simultaneously looks back to the great traditions and forward to an evolved future. It will take us along a path that is truly holistic, evolutionary, intentional, person-centered, and dynamic. We will learn how to undertake an integral assessment, design a program of integral practice, and progress toward integral health.

Finally, we will arrive at our goal—profound and enduring health, happiness, and wholeness. These achievements of integral health and life are of a different magnitude than what we ordinarily mean by these terms. Here we are speaking of:

- *Integral Health,* self-generated and self-cultivated, that leads to a comprehensive, holistic, and far-reaching healing of body, mind, and spirit and that is immune to life's adversities, including disease, aging, and death.

- *Authentic Happiness* that arises from within and is expansive, robust, passionate, and unaffected by the circumstances of daily life.

- *Genuine Wholeness* that experiences the interconnection of all life, a seamless existence and an uninterrupted oneness that is accompanied by ease, universal loving-kindness, and a lightness of being.

These achievements will bring us toward the highest and best that is possible for each of us. By reaching toward human flourishing, we become co-creators in the next evolutionary leap of health and healing. We continuously create more and better health for ourselves and for our world. Nothing less will do if we are to fulfill our human destiny.

I am now entering the third phase of my medical education—the most subtle, refined, and important aspect of becoming a better person and a more skilled healer. As I increasingly experience glimpses of the profound and enduring health, happiness, and wholeness that is possible for each and everyone of us, I simultaneously experience a deeply felt sadness that emerges with the recognition of the needless suffering and premature illness that are so pervasive among human beings. This heartfelt concern and care is slowly forging within my soul and spirit a compassion that I have long known is the only genuine motivation for becoming a healer. When one begins to know the gap between what is possible and the actuality of what is, inaction becomes untenable. Service becomes the only meaningful response. The arising of an authentic compassion and its call to service are the core of this third phase of my medical education.

It is my aspiration that the information and practices in this book, your personal reflections, and daily practice will help give rise to a profound and enduring health, happiness, and wholeness, and that these qualities of human flourishing will grow and ripen over time.

—Elliott S. Dacher
Crestone, Colorado
Dharamasala, India

The
Vision

This Precious Life

Imagine being taken on a special voyage to a treasure island. But at the end of your stay, you're unable to see the abundance of jewels everywhere on the island, so you depart empty-handed. How sad and disappointing that would be. Yet that is too often the unfortunate fate of our life. We live blindly among unimaginable treasures, and at the end of our days, we leave life unaware of the great wealth and the great health that have always been right in front of us.

What are these great treasures hidden from our ordinary vision? They start with something as simple and yet profound as being born into a human life. Eastern philosophy tells us that our chances of being born as a human are less than the possibility that a small, blind turtle living in an immeasurable sea can raise its head above water once every hundred years and place it through the center of a single golden ring buffeted across the sea by endless winds. There are more living creatures in a clod of earth than humans on our planet. To be born and live as a human is a precious and rare treasure. Yet there is more.

Unlike all other living beings, we are born with a unique and highly developed consciousness that endows human life with the capacity for language, creative imagination, self-reflection, discriminating intelligence, loving-kindness, and a good heart. If we choose to fully develop them, they enable us to realize in our lifetime an expansive and sustained flourishing of body, mind, and spirit. No other living being is endowed with these precious possibilities. We are destined for more than ordinary health or an ordinary life.

MOVING BEYOND ORDINARY

Even in the midst of our ordinary lives, most of us are given occasional subtle hints and quick flashes of what is normally hidden from us, tastes of precious health and well-being. Remember for a moment the first blush of romantic love with its ecstatic sense of peacefulness, openness, joy, and connection. This same glimpse can be experienced through a communion with nature, sacred rituals, the arts, sexuality, and athletic competition. In each case, we briefly touch an elevated state, but, taking it as a momentary high, we fail to recognize its greater significance.

These so-called *peak* experiences are really *peek* experiences—passing and partial glimpses of the great treasures of life and health. It's as if the longing of our soul for a profound wholeness and completeness is always pushing through in one way or another, giving us an occasional, tantalizing peek that seems unattainable and unsustainable in ordinary life. We grasp and cling to these momentary glimpses only to be quickly disillusioned when they invariably vanish as quickly as they arrived, dropping us back to ordinary health and ordinary life.

Although these glimpses offer us an opportunity to touch, taste, and briefly experience some of the profound qualities of a far-reaching health and well-being, we do not know how to hold or further develop them. In time, we forget them, discounting their significance and the possibilities they point toward, unconsciously betraying ourselves as we turn away from our highest and best possibilities. Instead of using them as a doorway to a more expansive life, we dismiss them as "weekend" experiences. A piece of our soul goes into hiding.

Now imagine the seemingly impossible: that you can stretch one of those moments out and at the same time profoundly develop, deepen, and sustain it so it is no longer momentary but rather your normal, continuous state of being. If this were so, you would enter into what is unquestionably the greatest adventure and discovery of a lifetime. Your life would be transformed. You would gradually realize the great treasures of human life. You would fully live the preciousness of human existence.

Does it seem impossible, just a fantastic fantasy? Can we actually have these treasures and riches, this high level of health and well-being? Look all around. Right now each of us is standing on a treasure island. Our capacity for a sustained health, happiness, and wholeness are right here within us, but we cannot see what is always and already there. We are standing empty-handed in the midst of great wealth, satisfied with a sliver of what is possible, thinking it's all there is, all that is possible. We are of the extraordinary, and yet each day we settle for the ordinary.

Like the butter hidden in milk, the flower lying dormant in the seed, or the gold encased in stone, human flourishing remains an invisible, unknown potential lying undeveloped within each of us. Although its potential is given to us at birth, it is hidden from ordinary view. Such health cannot be measured, analyzed, developed, or acquired in the usual ways associated with ordinary health. Nor is it a process of adding another technique or therapy, alternative or conventional, or another prevention strategy or psychological manipulation. All these efforts, these external remedies and self-regulation strategies, can improve our physical and mental health, but they cannot radically transform it. They cannot take us out of the box we are currently in. They cannot take us to another level of health. In fact, they delude us into a satisfied complacency and, in so doing, stop us from going further. Our fate becomes one of an ordinary life, an ordinary health.

MOVING TO THE EXTRAORDINARY

Integral health can only be known and achieved through the development of our inner life and our inner healing capacities. If we want butter, we must first know that it is hidden in milk and then learn how to churn milk. If we want a more profound health and life, we must believe in its possibility and then learn how to develop our consciousness.

The moment we start to seriously invest in growing our inner life and acquiring its natural healing resources, we simultaneously step out of our ordinary ideas about health and begin the climb toward the treasures at the summit of extraordinary health. We become increasingly free of the ravages of emotional distress and premature disease. And these disturbed mental and physical states are gradually replaced by a natural wisdom and loving-kindness that emerge at higher levels of consciousness. That catalyzes the development of an expansive health, happiness, and wholeness, which affects all other aspects of our life. In this way, a developing inner life transforms ordinary health and life into extraordinary health and life.

Each of us is given a sealed envelope at birth containing a map with instructions that can take us to a precious health and life. At several points in each lifetime, we are given the opportunity to open this envelope and discover its contents. Perhaps it is one of the glimpses mentioned earlier, or a brush with serious disease, death, or loss, maybe an unexpected moment of illumination and inspiration, or a persistent and unrelenting sense that there is more to life than we are living. Some of us will be profoundly and permanently moved by such experiences, grasp the opportunity, open the envelope, and begin down the path toward what were previously unknown and unimagined possibilities. Yet most of us will be too busy, too content, too quick to apply a remedy and diagnostic label to suffering, too preoccupied with the materialism of life, or too hypnotized by everyday existence. Caught in the perpetual cycle of day-to-day life with its alternating pleasures and pains, some of us will let this uniquely human opportunity slip away unnoticed. We will pass this unopened envelope on to the next generation, assuring ourselves of a "normal" life and ordinary health, leaving the deeper mystery and its treasures for others to ponder.

THERE IS NO TIME TO WASTE

There is a story about a fisherman who goes down to the sea one morning before dawn. He finds a sack filled with what appear to be small pebbles, and he proceeds to throw them one at a time into the water until the first light of morning. When he takes the last pebble out of the sack, he is startled to notice that it is a diamond. Mistaking the diamonds for pebbles, he has thrown all but one into the water. He was a lucky man. He still had a single diamond left. Most of us throw them all away. Our diamonds never look like diamonds at first glance. They are encrusted by ordinary rock until we polish them with the inner work of our life. So we unknowingly throw away all our diamonds—our potential for expansive and sustained health, happiness, and whole-ness—arriving at the end of our days without realizing or perhaps even imagining the essence of human life.

In this moment, today, right now, we have the opportunity to open the envelope and seek a comprehensive, far-reaching health and healing and a more profound life that is ours for the asking. As members of a highly advanced technological society, we have all the necessary outer and inner resources. We have a sound mind and body, our basic material needs are met, we have great freedom and far more leisure time than previous generations or people in other cultures. As a species, we have already devel-oped our consciousness from its most primitive instinctual patterns to a highly devel-oped reasoning mind. Scientific medicine has extended our life span and lessened physical pain and suffering. Most important, we now have access to the teachers and teachings that can enable us to attain integral health and life. We are primed to live our highest and best; we are ready to become fully human.

However, this opportunity will not last forever. When our minds have lost their superlative capacities through aging or disease and our bodies have become infirm, it is far more difficult to begin to pursue a more expansive health. Unseen, the promised and unique treasures of human life will slowly slip away. The hours of full capacity given to us in our lifetime are limited indeed. As a certainty, each of us will face death; the only uncertainty is its date and time. Perhaps it will be in fifty years or in the next hour. In either case, we have little time, and none to waste. Whether we are twenty or seventy, the time to seek the richness of human life and the fullness of health is now. Every moment spent occupied with limiting visions of health and healing and the simultaneous illusion that ordinary health is the best we can have takes us away from what is possible. If we are to fully unfold and live our precious possibilities, we must feel the urgency and, much as the alchemists have done, focus our mind's eye on finding the true unalloyed gold of an expansive health and life.

ONE VISION, EAST AND WEST

For most of us, this vision may seem like a far-off dream, a new-age fantasy, another variant of our unquenchable thirst for novel approaches to health. Or perhaps it rings true but seems too large to approach and too unreachable for now. But this is not so. Unlike a dream that we know upon waking is an illusion, this vision becomes progressively more authentic as we awaken to a deeper and more expansive consciousness. Unlike a new-age fantasy that lacks legs, or a novel approach that is usually no more than rearranging furniture in the same room, this vision is a natural and essential next step in the continuing evolution of human consciousness and in our progressively expanding capacity to heal the suffering of body, mind, and spirit. It is built upon a solid foundation that has been well prepared in the East and the West. It is neither unapproachable nor inaccessible. The essential ingredients are available. The methods have been mastered, recorded, and taught over many generations. There are many paths and practices to suit varied dispositions, and each of us can begin by taking small steps. A comprehensive and far-reaching health is a very real and achievable possibility.

In fact, it is the *traditional* dream of healing. The master healers in both the West and the East have continuously sought to reach toward the highest level of health. In the West that wisdom is fully expressed in the symbol of Asclepius, the Greek god of healing. In his right hand, Asclepius holds his famous staff that touches the earth and is encircled by a serpent. The staff signifies our connectedness to the earth, the elements, and the matter of life from which all external physical remedies arise. The serpent represents the inner wisdom that is the second great source of healing. It represents the more subtle remedy that extends beyond the physical to mind and spirit. The figure of Asclepius represents the fully conscious and fully developed healer within each of us who can properly weave these outer and inner aspects of healing into the richness of a comprehensive, fully integrated, and far-reaching health.

In the East, the mystery of healing has been expressed in the symbol of the medicine Buddha. In his right hand, the Buddha holds the Arura plant, which represents the power of external healing remedies. In his left, he holds a bowl that contains the healing elixir of inner wisdom. Traditionally, the bowl is a skullcap signifying the defeat of death. Similar to the figure of Asclepius, the Buddha symbolizes the enlightened being lying dormant within each of us who can comprehend, integrate, and apply these external and internal ways of healing. What we discover from these inherited symbols is that the traditional dream of healing, West and East, is precisely the same: expansive and perfected health of body, mind, and spirit attained through both outer *and* inner development.

FROM BODY TO MIND TO SPIRIT

So here is the challenge posed to us by the great healers. Are we satisfied with a normal life of seemingly relative ease and comfort in which we learn how to temporarily and partially minimize, console, and suppress life's sufferings through advances in modern medicine, prevention strategies, material gain, stress management, and other physical remedies and psychological techniques? Or do we wish to unfold an entirely new dimension of health and well-being, one based on the special glory reserved for the human condition? Do we wish in our brief lifetime to reach for the extraordinary treasures of this perfected life and health? "Tell me," asks the poet Mary Oliver, "what is it you plan to do with your one wild and precious life?"

In my twenty-one years of practicing internal medicine, I have observed and participated in the lives of many people, most often at times of acute and unexpected suffering and even at times of imminent death. What I have noticed is that each of us has different temperaments and capacities, allowing for different levels of consciousness and health. We are not all ready for larger health and life. Some are immersed in customary cultural perspectives. They view suffering, physical or emotional, as an unwanted intruder to be gotten rid of, managed, or suppressed as soon as possible. They look toward healers, conventional and alternative, to prescribe the most powerful external remedy that can be found. They believe the teaching of our culture: External agents are the only authentic sources of healing. Suffering may be diminished and perhaps even a cure may be attained, but there is no change in awareness, understanding, or ultimately health. There is merely the ongoing cycle of symptom, diagnosis, and remedy. Such is an ordinary health, an ordinary life, and an ordinary death.

However, some of us are able and willing to go a bit further. Here we may begin to look at the emotional patterns that underlie disease. This mind/body approach to healing recognizes the role of anxiety, stress, and other mental factors in the development, perpetuation, and recurrence of illness. As these factors are explored, it becomes possible to tailor a series of mind/body approaches such as psychotherapy, relaxation techniques, yoga, and biofeedback. These individuals are now able to increasingly experience the dynamic movement of mind and body, recognize their personal role in suffering and disease, and to an extent substitute internal remedies for outer ones. Self-reliance and personal competence are strengthened, suffering is diminished, and a broader sense of health is achieved.

Others of us seek a state of health motivated by an aspiration for something more, a positive state of well-being. Much as we have learned about the signs and symptoms of disease, we are now learning about the signs and symptoms of health. These include a sense of inner control, competence, and self-confidence, creating and sustaining healthy relationships, and having a sense of meaning and purpose in life. This expanding psychological health leads to more happiness and less distress. Here again new and more refined skills are learned, previously unseen capacities are developed, self-reliance is further strengthened, suffering is progressively diminished, and an even broader sense of health is achieved.

Finally, still others whose temperament, capacity, and circumstance are primed and ready for more, seek a level of health that is fundamentally and radically different from those described above. That can only come about through a leap in consciousness—self-transformation rather than self-regulation or self-improvement. Here we are no longer rearranging or adding furniture to the same room. We are now reaching toward profound and sustained health, happiness, and wholeness that embraces all we have achieved but at the same time is radically different from what we previously called health.

Such individuals usually reach this aspiration and possibility after traversing each of the preliminary stages described above. For them, the center of gravity of healing progressively shifts from physical to psychological to spiritual, from outer reliance to inner development. As we approach a more profound form of healing, the diagnosis of the causes of distress is more subtle and precise and the antidote or remedy is self-generated, comprehensive, and more accurately aimed at the source. With the insight of an expanded consciousness, we can now see what could not previously be seen. We discover with a certainty that needless suffering can progressively come to an end and that it can be replaced by an expanded life and health. At this stage, we are fully engaged in the broadest and deepest vision of health and healing, its understandings, methods, and practices.

We cast aside our self-imposed, limiting ideas as we step into our possibilities and claim for ourselves what is natural and proper for humankind. We are now poised to define health by what is possible rather than what is customary. In the process, we are taking it back from professionals and culture whose limitations have insidiously become ours as well. This effort requires no less than a profound leap in our understanding, capacity, and consciousness. This is what we are now called to.

The call to find a more profound health and life compelled this well-trained scientific physician to travel to a far-off land to sit quietly and study the wisdom of the great healers. It was in the East that I first heard a scholarly teacher and healer speak the words: "This is a precious human life—rare, treasure-like, and fragile." I must admit that I had to hear those words repeatedly over many months before I accepted them as my own truth. But it was not only the teacher's words; it was also his eyes. When he spoke these words, his eyes were deep and clear; with an undeniable certainty, they projected life's wisdom and offered its riches. In time, I came to know that this heartfelt recognition of the preciousness of human life is the first and most essential step on the path to integral health and life. For without this recognition, we will neither care enough about our life nor feel the urgency to let go of what must be given up in order to take on what must be taken on.

Once we hold the preciousness of life and the possibility of human flourishing near and dear, its remembrance no longer fades with the busyness of daily life. Then all thoughts, speech, and action begin to be measured by a different standard. Rather than patching together an ordinary life and ordinary health from the partial opportunities laid out by our current culture, we begin to demand more from ourselves. We are willing to set out on this new adventure in search of life's greatest treasure, the flourishing of human health, happiness, and wholeness.

To be a hero in our time is to journey toward the only territory that remains unexplored, the deeper more subtle realms of the human experience. Henry David Thoreau wrote, " . . . if one advances confidently in the direction of his dreams, and endeavors to live the life he has imagined, he will meet with a success unimagined in common hours. If you have built castles in the air, your work need not be lost; that is where they should be. Now put foundations under them." In the West and the East, the great healing dream envisioned access to the richest treasures of human existence. Encompassing both a traditional and a modern vision, we seek to lay a new foundation for health and life.

Consciousness and Health

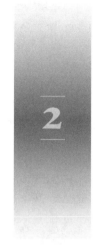

Every four years, we are amazed at the feats of athletic agility and endurance performed by the fully trained Olympian body. As we marvel at the far reaches of physical fitness, many of us are motivated to further develop our own fitness. Yet few of us have ever seen or known Olympians of the mind whose *mental* agilities and capacities are equally astounding. By redirecting their energy from an exclusive focus on outer things to a focus on inner development, they have attained Olympian mental fitness accompanied by a profound well-being of body, mind, and spirit.

What we are learning from these inner scholars is that the key to the next *quantum* leap in health and healing will emerge from the development of our inner life and our consciousness. In order to integrate the methods and practices developed by these mental Olympians, we must be willing to refocus our energy, attention, and efforts on exploring the still uncharted frontier of the human mind and its healing capacities. If we accomplish this, we can bring together the West's mastery of outer healing with the East's mastery of inner healing. The result will be the transformation of ordinary health into precious health.

It has only been recently that we in the West have become interested in the mind, consciousness, and health. In a sense, it was just yesterday that we became aware of the far reaches of mental fitness. The origin of psychology goes back a mere 130 years, biofeedback 50 years, developmental psychology 50 years, relaxation techniques 30 years, and psychoneuroimmunology 25 years. These efforts pale in comparison to the 2,500 years devoted to the exploration of consciousness and health by our neighbors in the East.

In a sense, the mind/body connection seems quite simple, and it is. We know that when we get nervous or upset, angry or agitated, we feel it in our stomach or bowel. This is a very old, commonsense understanding of it. Taking it a bit further, it can be said that underlying every ulcerated stomach, when carefully analyzed, is an ulcerated life—often filled with anger, painful aloneness, depression, and fear. And when our inner life is disturbed in this way, we also take our inner unrest into the outer world where it has an effect on our outer relationships and experiences. In this way, both the physical condition of our body and the character of our outer experience are strongly influenced and shaped by our state of mind. Our level of inner development cannot be separated from our physiology any more than we can separate ourselves from our shadow. We know from our day-to-day experiences as well as from newly emerging scientific research that consciousness and health are tightly interwoven.

ESTABLISHING THE
MIND/BODY CONNECTION SCIENTIFICALLY

The pieces of the puzzle have been coming together for decades, from the emergence of Western psychology to more recent neuroscientific studies of contemplative scholars. A good example is the field of investigation called psychoneuroimmunology (PNI) scientific exploration, which examines the relationship between the mind and the body's immune system. In the early 1970s, Dr. Robert Ader, Professor of Psychosocial Medicine at the University of Rochester and an early researcher in this field, achieved one of the first breakthroughs. Conducting a typical behavioral conditioning experiment, he fed laboratory rats saccharine-sweetened water mixed with a nausea-producing drug called Cytoxan. The rats soon learned to associate the drug-laced sweetened water with the nausea the drug produced. When Cytoxan was subsequently removed from the water, the rats continued to develop the symptoms of nausea even though the drug had been removed. The medicine was no longer the source of the nausea. That was now a mentally *learned* response triggered by the mere taste of sweetened water. It was all in the rats' mind.

Although this was of some interest, what happened next was of far greater significance. Within weeks, the rats began dying of infectious disease. What was happening? You need to know that the drug Cytoxan is an anticancer drug designed to suppress the immune system. So the important discovery here was that the rats' minds had learned to reproduce, without the actual drug, the suppression of the immune system much as they had learned to reproduce the nausea. The rats were capable of mentally altering their immune systems, something never before thought possible. The implications for humans that our consciousness could self-regulate this important guardian of our body are astounding.

At the Menninger Clinic in the early 1970s, Elmer and Alyce Green discovered that by using mental imagery, the mind can affect many of the physiological functions of our body. With the help of biofeedback machinery, we can train our minds to voluntarily control our blood pressure, pulse, muscular tension, skin temperature, bowel motility, and a host of other activities. Something as formless as a mental image, thought, or awareness itself can be translated into a physical experience. How was this happening? How was the mind speaking to the body? And how could this extend to the highly mobile immune system circulating in the bloodstream?

We already knew two ways that the mind and body interact. Each of these required "hard-wiring." The first is the autonomic nervous system, which controls the automatic physiologic mechanisms of the body such as our blood pressure and pulse; the second is the central nervous system, which moves our muscles when we choose. Each of these systems depends on hardwired nerve connections between the brain and the body. So how can our mind affect our mobile immune system when there's no hard-wiring hooked up to it? For the answer to that question, we had to dig deeper.

In the early 1970s, Candace Pert, currently a research professor at Georgetown University, filled in the missing link. She discovered a series of natural body proteins, called neuropeptides, that constantly circulate throughout our body, carrying messages back and forth. This was the third mind/body communication system, and a mobile one at that. These neuropeptides are made by many cells in the body and act on other cells and entire systems. The brain talks to the immune system, the heart to the kidneys, the glands to each of our cells and so on, creating in the process a fully interconnected community.

Even more important was the later discovery by Candace Pert and others that thoughts, feelings, and visual images—the stuff of our minds—can produce specific neuropeptides that alter our physiology to reflect a specific mental state. A mental event can lead to a physical event. Here was an important clue. If we could control, dissipate, and transform the negative emotions that occupy our mind, we could simultaneously reverse their deleterious effect on the body. Going even further, if we could transform our mind in the direction of health, happiness, and wholeness, our body would also smile. For this, we need to turn toward developing a rich inner life.

We are now witnessing the development of an entirely new field of neuroscientific research that is examining the relationships between the mind and the body. With our modern PET scanners, functional MRIs, and elaborate EEGs, we can see how mental activity—anxiety, depression, mood swings of all sorts, or, their opposite, a sense of well-being —can alter the blood flow and metabolic activity of specific areas in the brain and can perhaps even cause structural changes. Now we can finally understand why a nervous mind results in a "nervous" stomach, and how the rats' minds could affect, through neuropeptides, their immune systems.

This discovery caused Dr. Pert to say, "The mind is the body, the body is the mind." That's how it works. The condition of our body is a reflection of the condition of our mind. A disturbed mind results in a disturbed physiology. A healthy mind results in a healthy physiology. Something as formless and immaterial as a thought, feeling, or internal image can change the physical makeup of our body.

Building on this and other research, scientists who were studying human physiology began a host of clinical research showing how the immune and other body systems respond to the movements of our mind. They discovered how the loss of a loved one, marital discord, the stress of test taking, anxiety, depression, loneliness, helplessness, powerlessness, and essentially all disturbing mental activity are reflected in disturbed physiology. And when the mind is chronically disturbed, its shaping of our physiology becomes increasingly permanent and destructive to our health.

In 1998, Dr. Peter Schnall, currently Professor of Medicine at the University of California, published a research report in the *Journal of the American Medical Association*. This research explored how this works in the real world. He studied midlevel business managers confronted with a stressful work environment, a situation all too familiar to most of us. He identified the managers who suffered from "job strain" and those who did not. Job strain was the inner experience of too much to do and not enough time to do it—high demand and low control. Unable to find their way through this difficult circumstance, these individuals developed feelings of helplessness, powerlessness, and associated mental stress. But not all managers in this same circumstance experienced these feelings. Some undoubtedly saw it as a challenge and could summon the inner resources to deal with the workload. Only those who felt overwhelmed developed these disturbing emotions, which led to chronic hypertension and an enlarged heart. The unrelenting stress of negative emotions etched permanent changes into their baseline physiology and the structure of their bodies.

The deleterious effects of stress are not limited to the work setting. A simple example illustrates how we are constantly dealing with stressful circumstances in our day-to-day lives. Consider the telephone. The modern telephone routing system is an endless source of feelings of powerlessness and helplessness as it mechanically instructs us to push the telephone keypad even when we seem to be going to the wrong place and yearn to speak to a human. So many times, we want to slam the telephone down but can't. Instead we "slam" our physiology. How many other routine activities lead to feelings of helplessness and powerlessness? If we observe our life carefully, we will see that stress, almost unnoticed and taken for granted, has become a routine part of our life.

In the East, they say that our mental life can affect our body like writing on water, on sand, or on stone. A brief mental disturbance disappears rapidly from our mind and body. That is like writing on water with a finger. A more prolonged mental disturbance and its physical consequences remain a bit longer like writing our name in sand. But chronic stress, which to most of us goes unseen because we have become insensitive to it, results in a permanent reshaping of our mind and body that is as difficult to change as etching in stone. This relentless disturbance of our mind, which too often passes for normal, is the primary source of emotional distress and premature physical disease— or, for added emphasis, dis-ease. It works to ensure illness rather than to assure robust health, happiness, and wholeness.

That's why a healthy and developed inner life is an essential complement to outer treatments. Like pushing on a pillow and having it pop up in another spot, outer reme- dies and therapies, psychotherapy, stress-reduction strategies, relaxation techniques, drugs, and other behavioral efforts to manipulate our environment *appear* to tem- porarily resolve the problem, but invariably it reappears somewhere else in the body. These approaches do not go deep enough. They do not touch the sources and roots of our inner experience. They do not work with the deeper and more subtle levels of the mind and the mind/body connection. That is why a sophisticated and thorough approach to our inner life is essential. For true flourishing of body, mind, and spirit, we must go to the root of our mind/body ailments and permanently heal them at the source. This requires inner development.

THE SCIENCE OF OLYMPIAN MENTAL FITNESS

Although there is much we can attain by physical training and even fitness-enhancing drugs, there is a biological limit to physical fitness. However, there doesn't appear to be a similar mental limit to developing the qualities of the mind. The constraints on mental development are highly plastic and can in large part be intentionally removed. As a result, the mind appears to be capable of limitless development; in fact, we do not yet know its far reaches. Ultimately there will be a limit to the speed at which a human can run a mile, but, in contrast, the development of compassion may be limitless. Rec- ognizing the vast potential for inner development encourages us to further explore the relationship of consciousness and health.

Consider the following question: If negative emotions can be so destructive to our health, can healthy mental states and even "supernormal" mental states affect our health in an increasingly positive direction? Only recently have we begun to investigate this possibility and with it the dimensions of previously unimagined optimal health and flourishing of body, mind, and spirit.

The importance of our inner life in health, healing, and personal flourishing is now receiving attention and early validation from high-tech modern science. In the past decade, Dr. Richard Davidson began this exploration at the University of Wisconsin in Madison. For many years, Davidson, studying electrical brain activity and variations in brain blood flow and metabolic activity, mapped out the areas of the brain that become activated by negative and positive emotions. He accomplished this in two ways. First, he looked at the brain function of individuals who related feelings of well-being as compared with those who were disturbed by negative emotions. In effect, he was comparing those who saw the glass half full with those who saw the glass half empty. Then he studied the brain function of individuals who were shown a series of images ranging from happy to very disturbing. With this work, he was able to identify the areas of the brain that became activated by positive and negative mental states. His research showed that a certain area of the right side of the brain, the right prefrontal cortex, is activated by negative emotions, and a corresponding area of the left part of the brain, the left prefrontal cortex, is activated by positive emotions. At first glance, it appears that we have different brain centers for positive and negative emotions.

In fact, Davidson's research suggests that each of us is born with a certain temperament and disposition, a certain baseline ratio of left-to-right activity. Some of us are born with more of a disposition to see the glass half full and others to see it half empty; some of us have relatively more left-sided activation and some more right-sided activation. And at any one moment, depending on our inner experience, our brain can shift from one to the other. When we are happy or content, our left side will take predominance over our right side, and when we are experiencing negative emotions, our right prefrontal cortex will predominate. Davidson called this shift a "state" change as compared to a more permanent trait. In other words, such a shift is usually the temporary result of a particular experience. So although individuals will "light up" the healthy and happy left prefrontal cortex as a result of a pleasurable outer experience, they will in time return to their baseline disposition.

In July 2003, Davidson reported in *Psychosomatic Medicine* the results of a study done on a group of employees at a biotechnology firm who were offered an eight-week course in stress reduction and relaxation techniques. One group took the course while the other group was waiting their turn. The first group was evaluated before the course, immediately after the course, and then four months following its completion through written assessments of their emotions and anxiety levels, brain activity, and their immune response to the flu vaccine given at the start of the program. This group was then compared with the group that was similarly vaccinated for the flu but still waited for their course to begin.

Following the course and for another four months, the participants showed a reduction in anxiety and negative emotions and a corresponding enhancement of well-being when compared with the group awaiting the course. This shift in mental state was correlated with activation of the left prefrontal cortex associated with positive emotions. And when compared to the untrained group, the immune systems of participants showed a significantly greater, more robust response to the flu vaccination.

WE CAN TRAIN THE MIND

The study mentioned above shows that a training program for *beginners* that helps to develop a healthy inner life can immediately and for months afterward enhance their level of emotional and physical well-being and their capacity for health. We are discovering that our mental and physical life are not predetermined and fixed, and our capacity for health is flexible, dynamic, and expansive. Therefore, *we know that the mind is trainable and that robust health can result from the systematic training of our mind through planned, systematic inner development.*

Indeed scientific studies of mental Olympians are confirming just that. Davidson is currently conducting experiments with highly trained and skilled contemplative scholars who have made inner development their life's work. At the time of this writing, we only have the preliminary indications of the directions of this research, but these indications are revolutionary in their potential significance. Davidson asked highly skilled contemplatives to exchange their "cave" for the Western laboratory. Once hooked up to sophisticated technology, they were asked to enter into what for them were well-developed mental states such as boundless compassion or pure awareness. The level of activation of the left versus the right prefrontal cortex was carefully measured with electrical measurements and functional MRIs.

What Davidson is discovering is that these Olympians of mental fitness have levels of activation of the left prefrontal cortex, the site that correlates with positive emotions, which are way beyond those of the ordinary individual. They're "off the charts." Because the mind like the body is very plastic, this study proves the mind can undergo permanent change when properly trained. It can be transformed from the ordinary to the exceptional.

There are other intriguing clues based on these studies. While one of the scholars was in a contemplative state of pure awareness, a loud, sudden, startling sound was generated not far from his ear. The contemplative remained completely alert and aware of the noise. However, there was no evidence of a startle response in his facial muscles or an expected brain response. The contemplative maintained a sense of calm, balance, and inner peace, completely unperturbed. When asked for an explanation, he responded that he was at all times in the present moment so why would he be startled. Most people are startled when their mind is wandering and it's quickly jolted back to the present moment. Now if the contemplative could maintain an inner calm and stability in the face of such a disturbance, it might be possible for us to do so in a traffic jam. We just need to train ourselves to surf the waves of outer adversity rather than to drown in them. And since we know that the body follows the mind, our body can similarly become impervious to life's adversities.

Add to this a further intriguing observation. One of the contemplative states Davidson studied was compassion. The contemplative scholar generated a sense of universal loving-kindness for all people and a wish that everyone be freed from suffering or harm. Brain measurements done during this session indicated an unexpected activation of the motor cortex, the part of the brain that controls muscle function. The researchers asked the scholar for an explanation. His answer was thought provoking. He stated that when he is in a state of compassion, he is at all times ready to act to help other individuals who are suffering. That, he thought, was the reason for the activation of the motor cortex. His universal loving-kindness is instinctively ready to reach out to others. Imagine if everyone could realize this capacity and power. So much more would be possible for humankind.

Testing highly trained individuals with Olympic levels of mental fitness shows us that the far reaches of human flourishing can be explored by training our mind. Now we have the first scientific evidence that it may be possible to permanently transform our body, mind, and spirit. We can intentionally create an extraordinary leap in health and well-being that is far beyond anything possible with physical medicine alone. This can begin with as little as an hour a day—about the time it takes to train the body. Each of us can begin to experience a flourishing of our health and life from the onset of our inner practice, much as we begin to notice growing physical fitness after only a few weeks of working out at the gym.

Davidson and other scientists are beginning to lend credence in our modern age to the ancient recognition that the mind and the body are inseparable. We now know that it is our mental life, for good or for bad, that largely drives the character of our body's physiology. Only the further development of consciousness can take us to the next level of health.

We can see why the great healers throughout time and in different traditions around the globe warned us about the dangers of neglecting the inner aspect of healing. Only through a developed inner life can we identify and heal the inner sources of needless suffering and premature disease and discover and live an Olympian health. We are no longer *limited* to ordinary ideas about health nor to ordinary therapies and remedies. We can now use both inner and outer forces of healing to achieve a precious health and a precious life—a profound well-being that will become a permanent part of our life like an etching on stone.

Not only can our consciousness influence and shape our personal experience, but it also can impact others. The power of our mind can transcend physical space to affect the body, mind, and spirit of all those we touch. An optimal state of health can become a healing force that emanates from us like rays of the sun, penetrating everyone and everything we meet. Now we understand what the great masters of healing, East and West, knew from the very beginning: Inner healing and outer healing are the two essential healing forces available to humankind.

Aesclepian Healing

3

If consciousness is the force that drives sustained health, how can we integrate this inner capacity into our life and into our medicine? Twice in Western history, we have accomplished the difficult task of bringing inner and outer ways of healing into balance. The first was at the time of ancient Greece and the second in renaissance Europe. These were what we call crossover periods, times in which the previously dominant way of viewing the world was in decline and its opposite was on the rise. And for a brief shining moment, inner and outer ways of knowing and healing were in their proper balance and harmony. When this occurs, there is a corresponding flourishing of the arts, science, healing, and of human life itself. Having lived through five hundred years of exclusive focus on the outer way, we are once again on the edge of another crossover period.

None of us can fault the remarkable achievements in the modern sciences and medicine that have resulted in dramatic improvement in our life. Yet, when an exclusive way of viewing the world reaches the apex of its success, its limitations become increasingly apparent. When we deny one aspect of life, sooner or later we notice the price, personally and culturally, of our blindness. The Eastern cultures have exclusively mastered the inner life, but this has been accompanied by material poverty. We in the West have exclusively mastered the outer life but ended up with spiritual poverty. In both instances, achievement in one direction led to suffering in the other. That is why the East is now witnessing a rise in materialism, and the West is now experiencing a rising interest in the mind and spirit. In each case, the forgotten half of the human experience eventually reasserts itself as our life force continues to seek a balance of inner and outer that alone can lead to sustained health, happiness, and wholeness.

What would a healing process look like that honored and used both inner and outer ways of healing in pursuit of human flourishing? By traveling back to the golden age of ancient Greece to both study and relive the ancient practices of Aesclepian healing, we can see firsthand how this was done. And we can then distill from that experience the essential elements of profound healing that can serve our current personal and cultural efforts to move beyond our partial and limited approach to health.

HOW THE ANCIENT GREEKS PRACTICED INNER AND OUTER HEALING

Aesclepian healing takes its name from Asclepius, the Greek god of medicine. In fact, all modern-day physicians can rightly be called Aesclepians. The oath of Hippocrates taken at the time of graduation from medical school begins with the words, "I swear by Apollo, Asclepius, Panacea and Hygeia. . . . " However, I doubt few physicians know the rich heritage they are vowing to uphold. This truly holistic heritage of inner and outer healing has been lost in our preoccupation with outer ways of healing, but I believe it resides in the heart and soul of every practitioner, showing itself in those moments of frustration when we know there is more to health and healing than we have been taught.

If we needed healing in ancient Greece, we would have visited our local physician and on his referral, or perhaps that of our family or friends, we would have undertaken a journey to one of the many Aesclepian healing centers that existed from 450 B.C. to A.D. 300 throughout the Mediterranean region. Because we were going on a healing retreat, we would pack our clothes and essentials, say goodbye to our loved ones, and begin our journey, most likely by foot.

While on our journey to the healing temple, it is likely we would meet others who were traveling to or returning from it. Of course we would stop and ask about their experiences. What brought you to the temple? What was it like? And, most important, were you healed? We would listen carefully as they related their experiences, seeking a glimmer of hope in their story. Perhaps we would hear of a healing that would stir us with excitement and anticipation, offering us the possibility for a resolution to our own ailment or suffering.

After days of traveling, we would finally arrive at the gates of the great temple where we would be greeted by attendants who would direct us in the purification process required for entry to the temple area. Before entering the retreat and participating in a sacred healing process, we had to shed the mental remnants of our daily life. Through bathing, fasting, or other rituals, we slowly prepared ourselves, letting go of day-to-day life in order to focus all our energies on the inner and outer healing process that lay ahead.

When we were ready, we would enter the gates of the temple. At first, we might see a stone pillar, like the one that remains at Pergamum on the coast of Turkey, inscribed with two snakes whose faces meet at the center. This great symbol would remind us that here we would find the meeting of the inner and outer ways joined together in a whole healing. Perhaps we would linger a moment in contemplation.

We would then proceed straight ahead to the temple of Asclepius where we would offer a honey cake or some cheese to the healing god. What the Greeks were acknowledging with their offering was that to gain renewed health, something had to be given up, something had to change. You can't just rearrange furniture in the same room, take a pill, or undergo a treatment. Transformation, in the form of a thorough healing, required letting go of what was no longer working in life to leave space for comprehensive healing and renewal. And the offering and devotion to the god, which was an outward projection of the healer within, was an acknowledgment of and symbolic surrender to the more profound healing forces buried in our mind and spirit, unseen because they are as yet unknown.

Finally, with great anticipation, we would make our way to the dormitory, settling in for a stay that would only end when we felt revitalized, renewed, transformed, and healed. We did not go simply for a cure or a fix, but for an encounter with the healing god, the healer within, the deeper medicine. Leaving our dormitory, we would begin to explore the healing ecology that was at the heart of Aesclepian healing.

First we might wander along the paths and streets of the temple area, a ritual we would likely repeat each day. We would pass the lovely gardens, perhaps listen to roaming minstrels, and discover the beauty and serenity in the art throughout the healing site. The greatest sculpture of ancient Greece, the works of Phidias and Praxiteles were arranged for all to see. Then we might listen to the ongoing philosophical dialogues taking place in small informal groups, engaging the mind in self-reflective exploration of the meaning and nature of life. Beauty, truth, and virtue were all aspects of the good life and of a more profound well-being. Perhaps the next day we might shift our healing focus to the body and visit the gymnasium for a hot bath, massage, fitness activities, or athletic competitions. There was plenty of time for all these activities for this was the daily fare at the temple. The sole focus of our time was the subtle unfolding of a whole healing process that went far beyond treatment alone.

Each afternoon we might attend the theater. The largest theater in ancient Greece was at the healing temple at Epidaurus. Still intact and still the site of Greek drama each summer, this theater with its perfect acoustics presented the great dramas of Sophocles, Aeschylus, and Euripides. The ancient Greeks experienced the theater somewhat differently than we do. Today, we think of theater as entertainment, but at the Greek healing temples it was deep therapy. The Greeks were more personally involved and engaged in the performances. One day they might experience the story of King Oedipus, a tale of fate and destiny, suffering and salvation. Perhaps their distress or disease would lessen as they came to understand the deeper meaning of suffering and the usually unseen opportunity it offers for a deeper healing. Suffering, seen through the story of Oedipus and raised to a larger level of understanding, might become a potential doorway to human nobility rather than a mere source of despair, hopelessness, or helplessness.

Over a few afternoons we might see the performances of the trilogy of Orestia. Here we could experience lust, betrayal, anger, vengeance, guilt, and shame and see directly the cause-and-effect relationship between unhealthy, afflictive, nonvirtuous behavior and a disturbed and dysfunctional life. The capacity through reason and virtue to control the runaway mind with its chaotic and destructive thought patterns was seen by the Greeks as an essential element of the healthy life.

Then there is the great story of the courageous Odysseus who left his beloved wife Penelope to fight at Troy. Taking twenty years to return to his wife, Odysseus endured horrific adventures, each honing his wisdom and maturity until he could return home having heroically completed the journey of awakening. And meanwhile, waiting and waiting, Penelope undertakes her own journey, teaching us other lessons about wisdom, loyalty, patience, perseverance, and abiding love.

Perhaps we can try to imagine the inner examination inspired by these great dramas, the wisdom gained, the truth learned, the barriers overcome, and the gradual inner healing that drove the outer healing. Theater was just one experience that catalyzed ongoing self-reflection that continued day after day, intermixed with other activities at the temple. The multiplicity of experiences together formed a healing ecology of body, mind, and spirit.

Each evening we would don our sacred white garments and solemnly walk to the abaton, the sacred healing temple. Here, with others, we would leave another offering to Asclepius and ask the god to visit in a healing dream and then go off to sleep. Perhaps Asclepius would appear in a dream that evening or perhaps he would do so another night. If we had a dream, it was always possible that the understanding it contained was in itself healing or provided new insights into our circumstance. It is likely that the following morning we would relate the contents of our dream to the temple priest, who would then help interpret it and perhaps prescribe certain physical activities, nutritional programs, medicinals, the surgical techniques of the day, or whatever might be called for according to the dream.

Day after day, we participated in temple life until we completed the purpose of our visit. Then it was time to say goodbye to the retreat, and the vital healing ecology of temple life. If we were sufficiently wealthy, we might leave a testimonial to our healing etched in stone or written on parchment for others to see. Many such testimonials tell us of the broad range of distress and disease that were successfully healed at the temples. What we know for certain was that the healing was a through-and-through healing involving body, mind, and spirit. One such testimonial written in 350 B.C. reads as follows:

> Believe me men, I had been dead during all the years of life that I was alive. The beautiful, the good, the holy, the evil were all the same to me; such was the darkness that formerly enveloped my understanding and concealed and hid from me all of these things. But now that I've come here, I have become alive again for all the rest of my life, as if I had lain down in the temple of Asclepius and been saved. I walk, I talk, I think. The sun, so great so beautiful I have now discovered men, for the first time; today I see under the clear sky you, the acropolis, and the theater.

Then we would gather our belongings and begin the return trip home, meeting others on the way, this time sharing our healing experiences. When we returned home, we would integrate what was learned into our day-to-day life and participate in regular community activities to honor the inner healer Asclepius.

FIVE CHARACTERISTICS OF AESCLEPIAN HEALING

Aesclepian healing practices have much to teach us in our modern-day effort to revitalize and enhance the quality of our health and life. Although the ancient Greeks' understanding of consciousness was quite limited when compared to the understandings arising in the East and their outer healing skills were of course quite undeveloped when compared to our own, they managed to take the best they had and synthesize it into a remarkable process of integral healing. They found a way to live inner and outer at the same time and to work with great skill at interweaving the healing of body, mind, and spirit.

However, the ancient Greeks did not directly address the inner life. They did so through the external symbol of the god Asclepius. Statuary of Asclepius depicts the god's face with great softness, kindness, gentleness, love, and wisdom. Seen from today's understanding, the qualities and healing powers attributed to the god were no less than the inner qualities and healing powers that are at all times present in each of us and are directly accessible through inner development. Our consciousness has gained sufficient depth so that we can take back these projected healing capacities and own them for ourselves.

Aesclepian healing had five essential characteristics that are important for us to fully understand as we seek to revitalize our current approach to health and healing.

1. Holistic. Aesclepian healing was truly *holistic*. It covered the full scope of the human experience, encompassing the four aspects of human life: psychospiritual, biological, interpersonal, and worldly. Aesclepian healing touched upon each of these areas, incorporating a diverse range of experiences and relationships.

2. Evolutionary. Aesclepian healing was *evolutionary*. It encouraged individuals to awaken into a large world of possibilities. Evolutionary development is the step-by-step changes in our life that extend our knowledge, resources, and capacities. Each leap in our development unfolds a new and more expansive level of existence that embraces what came before and transcends its limitations. We are not stuck in one place; we are capable of moving from neutral to alive to more alive to fully alive and finally to human flourishing.

   Evolutionary change is driven by a progressive expansion of consciousness and understanding. It begins with a shift in consciousness followed by a shift in knowledge, priorities, and capacities. It is self-generated and self-cultivated. Such a thorough change is permanent and affects all aspects of our experience. We interpret, relate to, and experience life and its possibilities differently. Through evolutionary development, we ascend to a new level of existence.

3. Intentional. *Intention* is the faculty of consciousness that allows us to thoughtfully, carefully, and proactively determine our choices and carry them out. In humankind, this is a highly developed capacity, although it is not one that we always use. We have been deeply conditioned to react in patterned ways. In the early stages of human development, this was an efficient and predictable way of dealing with threatening circumstances. But we are no longer threatened by tigers in the bush. To deal with modern-day concerns and to look toward a future of human flourishing, we are required to develop and use this advanced human faculty.

   Intention is closely related to attention. We need to learn how to place and hold our attention on a chosen experience. If not, our attention will be automatically drawn to random thoughts, feelings, and images, and intentional choice will not be possible. Our capacity for intention and attention is refined through contemplative practice. When it comes to health and healing, these skills allow us to carefully choose and attend to our goals and priorities.

4. Person-Centered. Aesclepian healing was truly *person-centered care*. At the Aesclepian temples, individuals had the opportunity to explore diverse approaches to the body, mind, and spirit and were always trusted to find what was best for them, what was tailored to their nature, what met their specific stylistic and developmental needs. That is quite different from our current medicine, conventional, alternative, and integrative, which places the method, technique, approach, and professional at the center of healing. Did you ever wonder why when you see a conventional practitioner it is his specific therapy that you need. Or when you visit a chiropractor it is her approach that you need, or when you visit an herbalist it is his approach that you need? Why is it that our life is always seen through the lens of the practitioner and his or her practice?

    A practitioner who listens deeply to an individual knows that the person will in time reveal to you and to themselves the deeper sources of their distress and the specific type of healing that is needed. Each of us deserves to be seen and listened to as individuals who are unique in our temperament, capacity, orientation, and needs. Asclepius, the wise healer within each of us, reminds us that healing and becoming whole must at all times be person-centered, tailored to the individual.

5. Dynamic. At the Aesclepian temples, each individual had the opportunity to explore diverse approaches to the body, mind, and spirit and was always trusted to find what addressed the current needs and circumstances of the individual's life. Healing must always be a *dynamic* experience. It is ever-changing because we are ever-changing. Authentic healing and wholing is not a process with a generic one-size-fits-all diagnostic label and therapeutic intervention that remains unchanging over time. Our life changes moment to moment and day to day, and what is appropriate for our growth and healing one day may become an obstacle the next. To see healing as a dynamic process is to feel its aliveness and its vitality.

These five characteristics—holistic, evolutionary, intentional, person-centered, and dynamic—were the essential ingredients of Aesclepian healing much the same as they, in their matured form, will be the essential elements of the new, expansive modern-day approach to healing. We do not need to invent something new; we merely need to remember the wisdom of the past and update it for our time.

Now is the proper time in our journey through this book to further define the term *integral health*. Integral means complete, whole, and fully integrated. Our vision of integral health transcends the limitations of all our current approaches to health and healing. It offers a truly holistic and evolutionary approach. Its goal is far-reaching: a flourishing of body, mind, and spirit that when fully realized will lead to an expansive and sustained health, happiness, and wholeness for ourselves and for humankind.

The
Path

Integral Healing

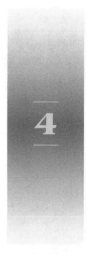

4

In the previous chapter, we explored the Aesclepian healing process and the five underlying principles that were the basis of this early integral approach. We are now able to go far beyond what was possible 2,500 years ago, or even in the past century. This is possible because of the momentous growth in our knowledge of science and consciousness. In its time, Aesclepian healing was an organic process that arose from the amalgam of tradition, myth, philosophy, and early science. Our contemporary approach to integral healing draws upon the modern-day wisdom and science of the East and West and relies on integral theory as developed by the modern philosopher Ken Wilber.

Integral healing is the proper approach for our time. It provides an important leap in vision that is equal to our current understanding and capacity, allows for an open-ended future, and assures a more encompassing health and life that go far beyond what is possible with conventional approaches. The integral approach is like a compass that orients and guides us toward an innovative and expansive healing process. It is distinguished by five guiding principles: *holistic, evolutionary, intentional, person-centered,* and *dynamic*. The first two are the core principles that define and distinguish the integral process. The final three are the application principles that guide us in applying the integral model to our life. The final goal of integral healing is human flourishing—a profound, hardy, and sustained health, happiness, and wholeness. Let's now examine the five principles that together provide a map to an integral approach.

PRINCIPLE 1: HOLISTIC

The integral map begins by simply acknowledging that the human experience expresses itself in four ways: psychospiritual, biological, interpersonal, and worldly. These four aspects of our experience are shown in Figure 1.

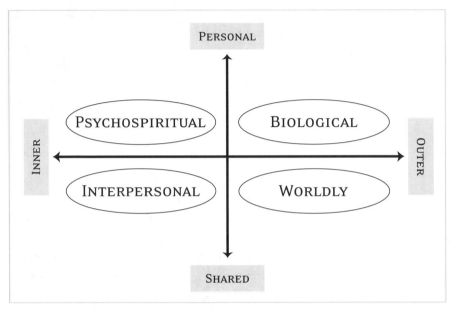

Figure 1. The Four Aspects of the Human Experience

Let's begin by taking a tour around the four quadrants of our integral map. On the right-hand side are the two aspects of life that we call outer: the biological and worldly. On the left-hand side are the two aspects that we call inner: the psychospiritual and interpersonal. The two top quadrants, the psychospiritual and biological, are personal areas of development. The bottom two quadrants, interpersonal and worldly, are the aspects of life we develop and share with others. This authentic holistic approach encompasses our inner and outer experiences and our personal and shared experiences. Each of these must be addressed when dealing with distress or disease and when striving for a more profound health and life.

These four aspects of life are interconnected. They are always impacting one another. An undeveloped psychospiritual life results in both a disturbed physiology and unfulfilled relationships. Disturbed relationships lead to a disturbed mental life and a disturbed physiology, and so on. It's like poking at a pillow in one place only to see it pop up in another. The integral map reminds us of these interactions and compels us to address each aspect of our experience. As a result it is truly holistic, fulfilling the first requirement of integral healing.

To make this a bit more personal, let's take a brief look at how each of these quadrants can make a difference in disease and in health. Let's begin with disease. Heart disease has a biological component that includes the narrowing of our coronary arteries, our diet, and our fitness level. It also has a psychospiritual component—a mixture of excessive stress, anxiety, and depression—and an interpersonal component—unhealthy relationships and low levels of social involvement. Finally, it has a worldly component: work stress, sedentary lifestyles, limited heart-healthy food choices, and in many instances, poor access to preventative health care. A comprehensive approach to heart disease must consider *all* these aspects of the illness.

With few exceptions, all our current efforts at healing disease and restoring "normal" health are limited to biological interventions—remedies, therapies, and energetic approaches located in the upper-right quadrant. This even includes our efforts to treat mental distress by simplistically reducing it to neurobiological abnormalities and treating it with psychoactive drugs. What is a four-quadrant problem is inadequately addressed as a one-quadrant issue. Because it is the misguided tendency of modern science to reduce life to its most outer expression and to ignore its other aspects, we are unable to fully heal or prevent today's epidemics of mental distress and premature disease, much less attain radiant health and life. To accomplish that, it is necessary to address all aspects of our life: each of the four quadrants. This requires an authentic holistic approach, an integral approach.

PRINCIPLE 2: EVOLUTIONARY

The unique genius of human life is our capacity to develop and evolve toward a progressively greater knowledge, complexity, and capacity. In each of the four areas of life, we can step up to a higher level of development that embraces our previous knowledge and capacity and at the same time transcends their limitations. With each step up, we acquire a more profound, accurate, and comprehensive knowledge of ourselves and our life. This shift, or we could say leap, is accompanied by new priorities, resources, and capacities. This unique human ability to evolve our life to higher levels of capacity and existence results from our ability for self-reflection, intentional choice, and focused action.

We can only develop and evolve potential that is already present within us. It is like the seed evolving into the flowering plant. The potential for this unfolding was always encoded in the seed, but the proper conditions were necessary for this potential to manifest—for the seed to realize what was previously a hidden possibility. So the full potential for a personal flourishing of health, happiness, and wholeness is present from birth, but we cannot know or see it until we have developed to a certain point.

Unlike the evolution of a species that occurs over vast periods of time and results from gradual genetic changes, the evolution of our personal life toward integral health is a result of conscious choice. It occurs as soon as we make and act on our choice. Through our choices, we can determine the extent and character of our development in each of the four aspects of our life. In this way, *we* determine the character and level of our health and well-being. Intention rather than biology is now the most pivotal factor in our personal unfolding. We can now assume authorship of our health and our life. Our understanding and use of this human capacity for conscious development and evolution is the second essential element of integral healing.

For example, consider your most intimate relationships, the interpersonal aspect of your life. When you look back on them, you can usually see a progressive development of maturity, capacity for intimacy, and depth. Less reactivity, self-righteousness, and defensiveness and a growing awareness, sensitivity, caring, and understanding of the other are signposts of this growth. As you gradually develop and evolve this aspect of your life, there is a corresponding expansion in your level of well-being that spills over and supports the evolution and development of the other aspects of your life. By developing your potential in this area, you are able to gain a level of health that was not previously present. This new level and quality of health are determined by nothing other than your choice and effort. As a result, not everyone will experience growth in this aspect of life. But it is possible for everyone.

In order to move toward integral health, it is essential that we value the potential for evolutionary development in each aspect of our life. We view our life holistically and then take a further step. We consciously choose to grow and develop our life in order to realize our full potential. To grow here and there as a fearful reaction to pain, suffering, or major illness is a slow, sporadic, inconsistent, and unpredictable process. Although fear may motivate us to grow our life, it will not take us to integral health. This requires conscious proactive choice. The integral map elaborates a blueprint for growth and development in each of the four aspects of our life.

Let's now take a look at this blueprint for growth and development in relation to each of the four aspects of life. It is important to note that I have chosen to discuss only four of the developmental signposts rather than fill in the many possible levels and sublevels of change. I believe it is more useful here to highlight the key levels of growth and development. So let's explore this second principle of integral healing.

The Psychospiritual

We begin with the personal areas of development—the psychospiritual and the bio-logical—because, in general and there are exceptions, our personal growth and development allow us to most effectively evolve our interpersonal and worldly life. As Gandhi said, "Become the change you want to see happen in the world." At this point in Western history, our psychospiritual life is our most undeveloped part, the primary source of the epidemics of mental suffering and premature disease and the greatest obstacle to human flourishing. It is the area of our life in which we can gain the most for our effort.

Just as a car needs a driver so does our life. Without the driver, the car could not properly arrive at its destination. Consciousness is the driving force that takes us toward integral health and life. It motivates, orients, and controls the entire process of human flourishing. When we develop our psychospiritual potential, our consciousness expands. Our level of consciousness determines the extent to which we can access our undeveloped potential. In this way, the development of our inner life is essential to all aspects of our life.

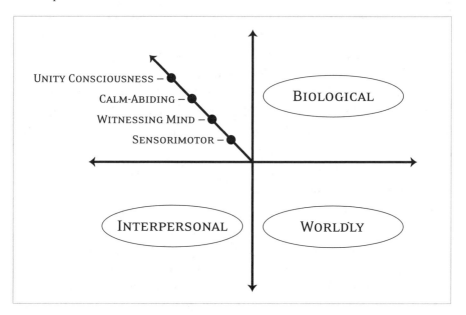

Figure 2. The Development of Our Inner Life

In Figure 2, I use the term *sensorimotor* as a baseline to indicate the most rudimentary form of awareness. You poke an amoeba and it knows to move away. From that rudimentary awareness, humans have successfully evolved many steps up the ladder of consciousness to arrive at the reasoning mind we have today. Our rational mind is responsible for the masterful discoveries and technologies of science and medicine over the past 500 years. It similarly guides us in our day-to-day life—organizing, planning, and directing our routine experiences.

The emergence of the reasoning mind was an extraordinary leap in human consciousness, capacity, and complexity. However, as we approach the apex of its achievements, its limitations become increasingly apparent. What we are discovering is that it is also the cause of many problems of modern-day life. It can neither reason us out of the modern-day epidemics of mental suffering and premature diseases nor can it bring us sustained health, happiness, and wholeness. For this we need to move to the next step on the psychospiritual developmental ladder, embracing yet transcending the reasoning mind in order to gain the new capacities we require to go further with our health and life.

The next major step shown in Figure 2 is the *witnessing mind*. To shift to a witnessing mind is to develop the capacity to step back and *observe* our mind and its thoughts, feelings, and images rather than automatically reacting to them. This is an extraordinary gain in control and freedom, offering a significant release from needless suffering. It ends our enslavement to the mind by creating enough space between a mental event and an automatic reaction to actually observe what is happening in our mind and to choose our response. When we develop the ability to observe our mind, we can end what seems like uncontrollable rumination. We save our energy rather than deplete it. The development of a witnessing consciousness offers us the ability to determine the character of our life rather than live unconsciously and reactively. This is an important leap in our well-being.

Developing the witnessing mind is accomplished through a series of exercises that help us tame and control the mind, thereby creating the capacity to witness its movements. We can then take actions that promote our health and well-being. We will discuss these practices in great detail in the following chapters.

Further growth in our psychospiritual life comes as we move to the next step in Figure 2 and gain access to the stillness of the calm mind. We call this level of development *calm-abiding*. When our mind abides in calmness, we gain openness, ease, connectedness, loving-kindness, and insight. We gradually lose the sense of isolation and separateness that is one of the fundamental causes of suffering and disease. We experience further health, happiness, and wholeness.

The final state of psychospiritual development, *unity consciousness,* is a pure and simple awareness. We have passed through the levels of psychological development and entered the spiritual life. This is an effortless state of clarity, peace, alertness, wisdom, oneness, and grace. These qualities spill into and spiritualizes all the other aspects of our life, catalyzing the movement toward integral health of body, mind, and spirit. Needless suffering comes to an end, our body returns to balance, and the yearning of our soul is realized. This achievement is a direct result of all our previous efforts. It ennobles human life by turning ordinary health and life into precious health and life.

This brief overview of the development and evolution of our psychospiritual life covers a great deal of territory. I have oversimplified a profound and complex movement for the purpose of demonstrating the breath and depth of what is possible.

The Biological

When we think of our body, it seems straightforward. But it is far from that, as Figure 3 shows. As an entering freshman in medical school, the first "person" we meet is a cadaver. We begin our exploration of human life by studying *anatomy;* this very basic, mechanical understanding is soon expanded to the study of *physiology.* Instead of solid immovable organs, we now experience a dynamic biology with all kinds of ongoing physiologic shifts and changes. This provides a far more complex view of the body that enhances our ability to treat illnesses and promote well-being.

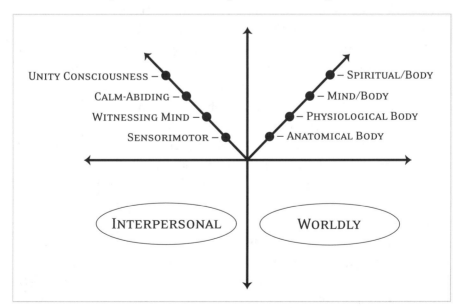

Figure 3. The Development of Biological Life

Medical education merely replicates what happens in our life. As children, we get to know the anatomical aspects of our body. We learned about our skin, bones, muscles, and limbs. We're told about our liver, heart, lungs, kidneys, and brain. It's only later that we learn about our physiology—our cardiovascular, hormonal, and immune systems. We're introduced to such concepts as high or low blood pressure, blood sugar, hormone levels, and digestive enzymes. We gradually realize that our body is vital and ever-changing. This is confirmed for us by laboratory tests that monitor the movements of our physiology and therapies that manipulate it. With this shift in understanding, we gain a more expansive, accurate understanding of our body. We are no longer just a collection of limbs and organs but vital, living beings.

This movement from the anatomical to the physiological body is embraced and transcended as we move toward an understanding of the mind/body. This next leap is a particularly difficult challenge for modern medicine. It requires a fundamental rejection of an exclusively biological view of the body. To embrace this shift is to acknowledge the role of the mind in health and disease. To fail to do so is to limit ourselves to partial health and healing. Many of us profess the importance of mind and spirit to health, but few of us act in accordance with this perspective in mind. There is a large gap between what we claim to believe and what we actually do in our day-to-day lives.

When our understanding of biological life evolves to include its relationship to the mind, we discover that the mind and body are neither separate from each other nor irrevocably set in place at birth. They are interconnected and plastic. Both these characteristics allow us to alter their function and structure through self-regulation practices. The body is no longer viewed as a fixed structure of organs with automatic physiological activities. It is now seen as a well-integrated information system that is constantly in flux and responsive to intention and proper training.

The discovery of our capacity to self-regulate our blood pressure, pulse, skin temperature, glandular secretions, and even our immune system through mind/body training was in itself a major accomplishment. But now we are going even further. We are learning how to reconfigure the circuitry of our brain. If we can fully develop and evolve this capacity, we will discover a previously unknown ability to co-create with nature the structure and function of our *mind/body,* thereby assuming a larger role in the self-cultivation of health and well-being.

At the far reaches of our biological and psychospiritual development, we view the body as the envelope of our immortal soul and spirit. Our perception of our body has undergone a dramatic shift from a physical body to a mental body to a *spiritual body.* We continue to embrace each of the earlier understandings of our body but transcend them by grasping a deeper truth—the knowledge that our physical nature is but an ephemeral expression of a far more vast and inclusive existence.

We know that we are simultaneously of the earth and of the stars, of the physical and of the spiritual. With this wisdom, we also come to know that death is a mere transformation from one life form to another. And this knowledge, attained through an evolved and expansive understanding of our biology and spirituality, softens our fear of disease, aging, and death. This allows for an ease and delight in life that was previously impossible. This is the movement of biological development from body to mind to spirit.

The Interpersonal

Having explored the principle of evolutionary growth as it applies to our psychospiritual and biological life, we can now see how these developmental steps influence the life we share with others. The wisdom and loving-kindness that we gain from our personal development affect both our interpersonal relationships and our worldly experience. This spiraling interactive process leads to a continuous outward expansion of our health and well-being.

The major growth in our interpersonal life is the shift from I to you to us to all of

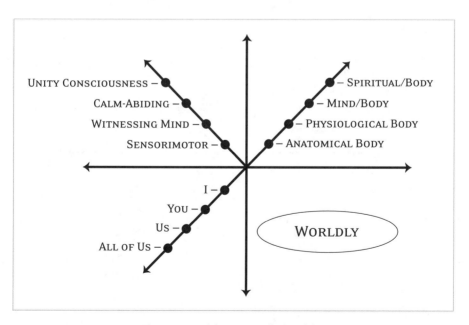

Figure 4. Evolving Our Relationships

us. From birth, we instinctively care for ourselves. In time, we come to see others as being as worthy and important as ourselves, beginning with our loved ones, then strangers, and ultimately even our enemies. With each step up the developmental ladder, our sense of isolation and separateness diminishes, and we gain a growing capacity for intimacy and connection. There is no longer a distinction between what we want for others and what we want for ourselves. In actuality, there is no longer I and other. There is only *all of us*.

We evolve our interpersonal life through a series of formal contemplative practices that we will cover later and through a conscious exploration of our day-to-day interactions. In this way we practice inside and we practice outside. Relationships are a major challenge. They force us to further develop our inner and outer life. We take on this challenge because they are central to our life. They bring us health rather than stress and joy rather than suffering.

Worldly Life

As we expand our consciousness and enhance our interpersonal relationships, we are better equipped to flourish in our outer life. A healthy inner life leads to a healthy outer life. Healthy personal relationships lead to healthy social relationships.

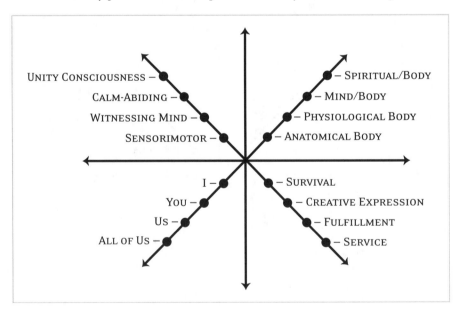

Figure 5. Transforming Our Worldly Life

An infant totally depends on the outer world for its physical and emotional *survival*. It cannot give to the world. It can only take from the world. The world serves our life rather than our life serving the world. This is how we relate to the world in our most undeveloped state. Unfortunately, this is how many adults continue to relate to the outer world. We persist in seeing it as a resource that we deplete to meet our physical and emotional needs. We act out of dependency rather than self-reliance, fear rather than confidence, scarcity rather than abundance. We neither flourish in our own life, nor does the world become a better place as a result of our presence. Even when we progress in our development we often retain the potential to reactivate this child-like way of relating. It can reemerge at times of stress and distress when we automatically look outward rather than inward.

As we progress in our development, the world becomes a place for *creative expression*. We begin to contribute rather than take. Our contribution may be in the form of a craft, skill, art, or other talent. We also contribute by expressing an increased appreciation for others, acting with loving-kindness and bringing care and compassion into daily life. With this shift in orientation, we change from an ego-centered use of the world to an active and meaningful participation in the world. Because we have more within ourselves, we can give more and take less.

We gradually realize that what we give to the world comes back to us as a renewed and revitalized sense of health, happiness, and wholeness. Previously, we mistakenly sought to fulfill our needs by taking from the world. Now we discover that our most important needs—the longing of our soul for meaning, purpose, and *fulfillment*—are actually realized through our full and increasingly selfless participation in the world. No longer is the inner world our sole source of peace and ease. Increasingly, as the distinction between our inner and outer life begins to blur, our worldly life—activities and people themselves—become a source of nurturance, development, and happiness.

Over time, our egocentric tendencies continue to soften. Our mind stills and our heart opens. It is no longer possible for us to turn away from the needless suffering in the world. We begin to see *service* as the most meaningful expression of our life. We discover that giving, caring, nurturing, and mentoring fills our life with health, happiness, and wholeness. We become a source of wisdom and loving-kindness for family, coworkers, and our local and global community.

We create in culture what we have created in our life. We seek to infuse wisdom and compassion into the institutions of culture—into our schools, governance, environment, healthcare systems, and social policies. Our aim is to participate in creating institutions of wisdom and compassion that will thoroughly transform our culture. We feel a universal responsibility toward all that is. Service then transforms itself into a sacred calling. We care for all of life because we know it to be inseparable from our own life. When we heal the world, we heal ourselves. We flourish and the world flourishes with us.

A wonderful example of what's possible in a spiritually based culture is the Gross National Happiness project of the small country of Bhutan. As an alternative to measuring the success of a culture by economic growth, the Bhutanese decided to measure the happiness of their citizens. They identified four social initiatives that most affected the health and happiness of their people; economic development that balances material needs with other social needs, sustainable environmental development, social services such as education and health care, and good governance. A report on their efforts in the October 4, 2005, science section of The New York Times shows that the spiritual and interpersonal development at the core of their religion and education has flowed into their political, economic, and social life, allowing for similar growth in their cultural life. I have included a website address in the Resources Guide that will take you to a variety of papers detailing this well-considered integral program for inner and outer flourishing.

These first two principles, the holistic and evolutionary principles, define and distinguish integral health and healing. The final three principles are the application principles. These three show us how to apply this approach to our life. We do so by using our capacity for intentional choice and action, by addressing our unique needs, and by responding to our life in a vital and dynamic way.

PRINCIPLE 3: INTENTIONAL

Intention is the mental ability to consciously choose and act. Without intention, we cannot direct our life. We are all familiar with the use of intention in our daily life. When we need groceries, we go to the store. When we're sick, we go to the practitioner. But much of our life is reactive and automated rather than intentional. Consider the following. Close your eyes for a moment and notice how your attention is involuntarily drawn from one random thought, feeling, or image to another. Do you notice how your mental activity is dictating where your attention goes? How much of your day is spent unconsciously reacting to what arises in your mind? When this occurs, where is your attention? Where is your choice? Too often, we blindly follow our mental activity rather than exert choice. Observe this for yourself.

Intention is essential to integral health. Without this capacity, we cannot choose to shift our focus from a conventional approach to one that is holistic and evolutionary. We cannot choose a new and broader vision of health, determine how to actualize this vision, and apply effort and perseverance toward carrying out the necessary activities. Any activity that breaks with our usual patterns must be initiated and carried out with conscious intention. That is a unique human ability. We need it to leap to the next level of health.

PRINCIPLE 4: PERSON-CENTERED

The fourth characteristic of an integral approach is its focus on the individual—on you and me. That means removing professionals and their therapies and remedies from the center of the healing process. Health and healing must address the needs of the individual rather than the approaches and perspectives of the practitioner. Each of us is born with a different disposition, style, temperament, set of capacities, and perhaps even a different way of approaching life's journey to integral health. We also come from different cultures that offer unique developmental pathways to steer our growth and development in the four aspects of life. What is correct for any one person at any one time may be quite different for another.

What steps must we take right now toward integral health and life? Which aspect of our life is the proper one to work on at this moment, given our age, life circumstance, level of development, capacities, and so on? Is it a time to rest and sit still or a time to be more active? Is it a time to begin contemplative practices, explore the difficulties in our relationships, attend to our psychology, work on our body, unfold our creativity, or grow into a family? Should we attempt one or more? Once we view ourselves as central to the healing process, we can then tailor a unique approach to integral health that is in accord with our specific needs.

PRINCIPLE 5: DYNAMIC

Respect and concern for the dynamic and vital movement of our life is the fifth and final principle. With an integral approach, we always consider the circumstances of today and act accordingly. This does not mean that we are constantly running from one thing to another. It means that we maintain a profound respect for the active flow of our life and sensitivity to those aspects of our experience that are calling out for healing. We must learn to stay the course when needed and shift direction or emphasis when that is called for. The integral map is just a map. It is there merely to remind us of the great mystery that is unfolding in its unique way in each of us. It is not intended to be a substitute for the living experience.

Each time I sit with an individual, it is an entirely new experience. I listen carefully in a community of truth neither imposing a particular approach nor seeking a specific diagnosis. I am seeking only to hear the essence of this individual's life and to allow his or her destiny to slowly emerge from the narrative. Every good healer will tell you that if one listens long enough and deep enough, the individual will in time tell the healer specifically what the problem is, the aspect of his or her life that now needs attention, and the unique way to approach this issue in this person at this time. It is never the same. There is no such thing as a generic diagnosis or a one-size-fits-all approach. Every life is precious and unique.

THE FIVE GUIDING PRINCIPLES

The five principles that characterize integral health distinguish it from all other current approaches to health and healing, which, by comparison, are found to be partial and limited. These five principles underlie and guide the full development of each of the four aspects of our life, placing us on the direct and proper path to human flourishing. With an integral approach, we learn how to move with confidence and clarity toward genuine and sustainable health, happiness, and wholeness.

Human flourishing is an opportunity. No one can do it for us. We must choose it for ourselves. If you choose to take this opportunity, the teachers and the methods will become available to assist you in this noble journey. What I have shared with you in this chapter is a map. I encourage you to take the journey it outlines.

Preparing the Ground

5

The path to integral health begins with specific preparations. These serve two purposes. First, they require a firm and genuine commitment to rechannel one's energies inward. Second, they prepare us for the psychospiritual practices that are essential to initiate the inward turn and the integral process itself. This is where our commitment and intentions are first challenged. It is where we begin to "walk our talk." Our emphasis shifts from vision to practice, from an intellectual foundation to the actual embodiment of integral health. This shift can only be done by ourselves, through our own choices and actions. These preparations will test the seriousness of our commitment. We begin to put vision and theory into integral practice by undertaking the preparations.

A seed requires the proper soil for its germination. If we plant it in clay or sand, it will not grow, but if we plant it in rich earth that is continuously cultivated, a beautiful garden will naturally arise. To gain full access to the possibilities of integral health, we similarly need to prepare a proper set of conditions. At birth, we can only reach out to meet our need for survival. With conventional education, we learn about conventional health care, treatment, prevention, and health-promotion strategies. But as we become sophisticated adults, we develop the capacity to consider, choose, and realize a more expansive integral health. For this possibility, we need to shift our priorities, cultivate the ground of our life, focus inward, and expand our consciousness. With these efforts, the seed of integral health can fully bloom.

Make no mistake: This turn toward inner development and integral health does not mean we have to turn away from the responsibilities of our outer life or the wonders of Western medicine. What we are turning away from is very specific. It is the *mistaken belief* that our worldly efforts alone can place us on the path to a sustained health, happiness, and wholeness. What we are turning toward is the *correct understanding* that the development of our inner life and an integral approach is the essential next step on the road to human flourishing.

THE PREPARATIONS

At first, we need to have faith that will motivate us to rechannel our energy from the exclusive pursuit of outer health and healing to a holistic and evolutionary integral approach. We accomplish this by reminding ourselves again and again about the unique and precious opportunities of human life, especially of our life. Next, we choose to cultivate an attitude of loving-kindness. Loving-kindness opens the heart and ensures the help and cooperation of others. This attitude then motivates us to become as skillful as possible in using our speech and actions to minimize disturbing outer experiences that cause distress for others and similarly agitate our own mind, leaving little space for our inner life to develop. Finally, we must strive each day to create an oasis of silence and solitude that will allow for contemplative practice to support and enhance the entire process. With these preparations underway, we can begin integral practice.

In the beginning, most people underestimate the critical importance of the preparations, preferring to rush on to the "real stuff." *But this is the real stuff.* I cannot stress that point strongly enough. To undertake these preparations with intention and a sincere heart means we immediately begin through our daily choices to rechannel our energy in the direction of integral health. These preparations are life-changing commitments in themselves. They cannot be bypassed. The wise ones who have already taken this journey—whether they be religious figures, philosophers, or scholars in both East and West who have achieved a deep sense of wisdom—have given us a record of their travels, and it always begins with these efforts. They knew from experience that we must carefully and properly prepare our life in order to embody a higher consciousness and expansive health.

As we slowly gain confidence in these initial steps, our efforts to develop and evolve integral health will accelerate in a very natural way. These preparations will continue to grow in importance as we progress. At the beginning they cultivate the proper foundation for our journey, in the middle they nourish what we have accomplished, and in the end they help to sustain our achievements. They are essential at every stage of our inner turn.

PREPARATION 1: LOVING-KINDNESS

Nothing can more effectively stabilize our mind and lessen the grip of self-centeredness than the embrace of others. This is our most powerful antidote to destructive emotions like anger, intolerance, jealousy, pride, and greed that agitate our mind and make it unavailable for further development. We each know the pervasive inner peace that arises when we embrace our beloved. Can we imagine the possibilities if our embrace became more universal?

All of us have experienced at one time or another profound kindness, compassion, and love for another person. Usually this is someone dear to us, a family member, lover, friend, or mentor. In order to show loving-kindness to others, we must begin by showing it to ourselves. We cannot give to others what does not yet exist within ourselves. So we must turn this loving-kindness inward. Next, we show it to those who are closest to us. We practice opening our hearts with kindness, care, patience, and generosity toward their needs.

Loving-kindness can be expressed in our thoughts, prayers, and advice or through physical assistance and generosity that connect heart-to-heart. Loving-kindness includes sensitivity and openness to others and their differences, a warm heart, and the qualities of respect, fairness, honesty, patience, and acceptance. If we look very carefully, we may notice that these were always our natural intentions toward others before self-concern took center stage. Like clouds moving across a clear sky, our loving-kindness is all too often obscured by our calculating mind that assesses the cost to ourselves. Then our kindness, generosity, and care are reconsidered and modified to suit our ego needs. Our open heart is compromised by the thinking mind.

We would agree that everyone, not just our loved ones, wants happiness and wishes to avoid pain and needless suffering. In this sense, every human being is equal to everyone else. Although many may strive for these goals in mistaken and even destructive ways, nevertheless we all seek the same thing. And why shouldn't every person have happiness and be free of pain and unnecessary suffering? Here again we're all in agreement. When we can see that everyone wants happiness and love, we can then move one step further and wish this for others. The final step in the development of loving-kindness becomes the simple aspiration: "I want to assist others in alleviating needless suffering and gaining happiness."

It is important to remember that we are referring now to the early preparations for our integral journey so it will suffice to develop the mental attitude of loving-kindness even if at this moment you are unable to take outer actions. The mind drives our outer actions so the mind is where we must begin. The point here is to cultivate the intention to shift our mental attitude from self-centeredness to cherishing others. When this inner attitude is sufficiently stabilized, we can begin to practice loving-kindness in the outer world.

It is important to remember, however, that self-centeredness is very deep and tenacious. It will take time and endless patience to completely overcome it. So we begin in little ways each day as we continue to work on this inner shift. It will not take long to realize that loving-kindness toward others can place us firmly on the road toward our own health, happiness, and wholeness. This is the advice of all the philosophical and religious traditions and of the great sages who have carefully considered the essentials of well-being.

PREPARATION 2: SKILLFUL ACTION

We begin this preparation by what at first may seem like an unglamorous step: learning to restrain unskillful behavior and encourage skillful behavior. By "unskillful behavior" I mean behavior that creates an obstacle to our inner development. Our aim here is to cultivate behavior that supports integral health and abandon behavior that produces obstacles. This is not easy for those who consider any control or discipline over their behavior as an assault on personal freedom. But, in fact, most, if not all, of our actions are highly conditioned and programmed, and few, if any, are actually freely chosen. What we aim to do here is to bring an end to destructive knee-jerk reactive behavior by becoming increasingly aware of its negative effects on our ability to still and calm the mind. We want our mental attitudes, the actions we take, and the character of our speech to support our inward turn and our efforts toward integral health.

All the great healing traditions speak with a single voice when articulating this message: If we seek to achieve the aim of life—deep and sustained health, happiness, and wholeness—we must begin with ethical and virtuous behavior. Spiritual teachers tell us that without this foundation, it is not possible to achieve sustained well-being. Anger breeds anger, violence breeds violence, hatred breeds hatred, covetousness breeds covetousness, and it all breeds an agitated and unworkable mind. Skillful behavior toward others, even at first when it may seem tedious and forced, is essential. It may be easier to lash out, close our heart, or behave impulsively, but we must remember that in the end we suffer from these actions more than anyone else, as they are concrete obstacles to any forward movement toward integral health. This is no moral statement, but rather the honest recognition that certain actions inevitably lead to certain consequences and that we must stop doing what hurts us before we can move forward.

There is an important principle that may help us understand the process and importance of the shift toward skillful action. Like hot and cold or wet and dry, opposing positive and negative emotions or positive and negative actions cannot simultaneously exist in the same moment. By enhancing what is wholesome, we automatically decrease what is unwholesome. As our afflictive emotions and behaviors diminish, the qualities of well-being become more firmly rooted in our life. This frees up energy for integral practice.

I often deal with this in my work as a mentor and counselor for individuals and couples. My clients can only begin their real work when they are out of crisis mode and cease creating problems for themselves and others. That is most apparent when couples continue to act out toward each other while sitting on the couch in front of me. They need a ceasefire. We all need an inner ceasefire. But we can't do that all at once. It requires constant awareness, strong motivation, and an ongoing focus on our final goal of human flourishing.

The three gates through which we act in the world are our body, mind, and speech: the actions we take, the content of our thoughts, and the character of our speech. So it is important to know what constitutes skillful action and what constitutes unskillful action, what cultivates an inner life and what obstructs it, what cultivates distress and what cultivates health. When we are about to act in a manner that is unskillful, we need to consciously choose restraint, and when we are about to engage in skillful actions, we need to encourage them. This requires an active vigilance and mindfulness as reactive patterns are quick, tenacious, and many times deceptively subtle. And when we are not perfect, which is most of the time, we must strive to learn from our actions rather than judge them.

Usually there is very little space between afflictive thoughts, feelings, and images arising in our mind and the immediate and automatic actions and speech that follow. Our negative energy goes out to the world, and then we have to deal with the backlash to our actions. Whether we're expressing fear, anxiety, anger, greed, jealousy, or insecurity, the pattern is much the same. Our life is too often like an out-of-control car without a driver. We must put the driver back behind the wheel in order to control the outward expression of disturbing thoughts, feelings, and images. That is why discipline and restraint are needed. Without them, we cannot grow our inner life, and without growing our inner life, we cannot attain integral health.

It is important to recognize that we can abandon behavior that is detrimental to our life. Fortunately, what is learned can be changed. But because certain inherently destructive behaviors may occur automatically and in the initial stages may even appear pleasurable—for example, feelings of anger and revenge—the decision to restrain them will at first require discernment and discipline. But with experience, we soon realize that destructive behaviors, however pleasurable they may seem at first, destabilize the mind, preoccupy it with mental chatter, and insidiously destroy our ability to develop an inner life. These temporary pleasures are in actuality self-satisfying self-betrayals of our potential for integral health and life.

I have personally found the distinction between skillful and unskillful behavior to be very helpful. It has encouraged me to measure my choices by several criteria. Do my attitudes, words, or actions take me toward my goal of integral health and life or not? Is my behavior self-serving, or does it serve others? Have my words or actions caused suffering or relieved it? Does the way I live my life support the oneness and wholeness of all of life or not? These have become the criteria by which I judge the appropriateness and skillfulness of my attitudes, speech, and actions. So I am now able to see my behavior as a tool that I can consciously and skillfully use to either place my life on the road to integral healing or take me away from my goal. I choose to be a master craftsman with my life. You can, too.

PREPARATION 3: SILENCE AND STILLNESS

Having opened our heart and mind with the previous preparations, we can now begin to focus on the value of silence and stillness, which is our most important doorway into a larger consciousness and integral health. This may turn out to be a major, and at times difficult, shift, but it is made far easier by the previous preparations. There are three aspects of silence and stillness: the outer, the inner, and the innermost. The latter two are progressively attained through mind training. The first refers to our outer condition—to the stillness and calm of our physical environment. The second occurs when we achieve an initial calming of the mind. The third arises when our mind effortless rests in its natural state of peace and ease, immune to the ebbs and flows of life's adversities. Our final preparation begins when we carefully examine our day-to-day activities and physical environment with the aim of identifying and eliminating sources of excess noise and busyness.

Reordering our life in this manner means toning down outer activities. It means letting go of what is unnecessary, trivial, and noise-producing, while actively seeking spaces of silence and solitude each day. Carefully examining our day-to-day life is an important step in identifying the factors that support the development of our inner life as well as those that serve as obstacles. We need to ask of each activity each day: "How does this affect my mind? Does it cause inner peace or a more agitated mind? Is it an essential activity, a needless distraction, or merely an amusing entertainment?" The choice is then yours—whether to embrace the activity or abandon it.

Consider the issue of noise itself or, perhaps, the activities that keep our mind buzzing all day. There is the telephone, television, newspapers, e-mail, radio, and all other kinds of outer communication that fill our mind with endless mental chatter, most of which is of little value to our life. It robs us of a quiet innerness. Or consider our conversations, social engagements, and other forms of entertainment, all of which similarly serve to keep our mind busy but in the end often leave us with nothing of sustaining value. Can we reduce or eliminate unnecessary activities that merely feed our mental chatter and occupy us in endless busyness? Can we let go of trivial conversations, unneeded entertainment, and meaningless social interactions? Can we distinguish between what feeds an inner solitude and what feeds a chattering mind? Do we know the difference between what is necessary for our life and what we are accustomed to think is necessary? Do we want a life of busyness or meaningfulness? You will be amazed at how much time and inner space can become available for integral practice when you shift your priorities.

This does not mean you have to assume a monastic life. In fact, it is our unique challenge in the West to learn how to turn toward integral health in the context of worldly life. At first this may seem difficult, if not impossible. But when our focus shifts from outside to inside, many activities we once cherished and deemed important will gradually lose their appeal, and in time they may even become undesirable. We will find that many of our outer activities that seemed essential merely served to temporarily and unsuccessfully fill an inner uneasiness. This, we discover, can best be filled by a daily oasis of silence and stillness rather than medicating our unease with ceaseless busyness.

As our inner life takes hold, we will find we participate in fewer activities, but those we choose will be more meaningful. Our friendships will diminish in number, but they will increase in depth. We will spend more time alone, but we will feel filled rather than lonely. In this way, we will naturally discover that our new priorities lead us toward a simpler, quieter life.

Renunciation is what we're referring to. This word is often a very uncomfortable one for Westerners. But renunciation here means nothing more than cultivating what brings us happiness, health, and wholeness and abandoning what keeps us stuck in stressful and unproductive life patterns. It means prioritizing and taking charge of what we truly want in life. When we see the truth of our life, renunciation becomes effortless and even desirable.

We renounce things all the time—things we don't like. So as we turn toward and begin to experience the blessings of an inner life, we will naturally turn away from many activities that, when seen from this new perspective, are now dissatisfying rather than pleasurable. A new clarity from within will unveil the truth that will allow us to more correctly see that these seeming pleasures were mere distractions from and obstacles to integral life and health. The wise guides from the past have always said that what we call happiness from outer pleasures, they call suffering. When we realize this truth, renouncing outer obstacles to integral life and health becomes a natural inclination.

So begin your search for stillness by taking an inventory of your life. Examine each aspect of your daily life with the singular question: What supports and what detracts from the development of inner stillness and silence? It is helpful to begin by making a list of those outer activities that are essential to your most cherished worldly responsibilities. Then list those that are of questionable value and finally those that are unnecessary and serve only to entertain or distract you. Begin by letting go of the unnecessary activities and slowly work your way to the marginal ones. It's like cleaning out a house room by room when we are about to move, letting go of unneeded things first. Start by identifying and then reducing or eliminating one unnecessary outer activity a week, and then use this liberated time for the practices described in future chapters.

Once your efforts are underway, old friends may go, new like-minded relationships may bud, activities previously thought essential will drop away, and more time will be spent alone. As our inner life takes root, aloneness will become a cherished source of peace, ease, and inner transformation. Letting go of what no longer serves you and taking on what supports your inner growth may not please everyone you know. But adjusting our life over time to allow for more inner stillness and silence will, along with the other preparations, cultivate the ground of our life so that the seed of integral health can fully bloom.

A VISUALIZATION: MEETING ASCLEPIUS

Know that it is the wise healer who resides within each of us who will help guide us through the preparations and the integral process itself. That wise one the ancient Greeks called Asclepius. It is now appropriate for us to visit our inner healer as we begin our journey toward integral health.

Find a comfortable seat, close your eyes, and visualize the image of a very wise, loving man or woman. Choose an individual, alive or passed on, whom you respect and honor and with whom you feel a special sense of connection. If identifying or choosing such a person is difficult, then simply create one. Stabilize this image in front of you and notice all the details about the person. Sit in communion with this wise person and feel his/her presence. Reflect on his/her qualities and characteristics, her/his peace, wisdom, compassion, love, and joy. The image of this individual should now become your focal point. Stay with this image and allow the experience to deepen.

When the image has stabilized in your mind, allow a strong beam of white light to form at the crown of his/her head. Next, allow the dense white light emanating from the mind of this wise person to enter into your mind. Allow this energy to bathe and purify your thoughts, feelings, and images. Slowly transform your mind into the mind of this person. Take all the time you need for this transformation to fully evolve.

Next, allow another beam of light to form and emanate from the throat of this wise person. Allow this energy to bathe and purify your speech. Take on the qualities of loving, wise, and sensitive speech so that yours becomes the speech of this wise person. Again, take your time as this transformation and purification take place.

Then, let a final beam of light emerge from the heart of this wise person. Allow it to enter your heart. Let it bathe and purify your heart with kindness, love, and compassion, transforming it into the heart of this wise person. Take your time in allowing this transformation to take place.

Experience your mind, voice, and heart as you take on the qualities of the wise one. Become this person.

Next, allow the entire image of this wise person to dissolve into a bright white light. Allow this light to enter your body at your forehead and slowly permeate your entire being, from your cells to your organs, so that you fully become this wise person. What does this feel like? What will it be like to have the wisdom and support of the wise inner healer assist you in your integral journey? For the next few moments, experience what it's like to be such a person, to be able to accept yourself as a wise and loving healer in body, mind, and speech.

Hasn't this possibility—this self—always been within you? Why is it easier to see this wise and pure aspect of yourself externally in another person rather than recognize it as your essence? Who is this wise and caring person you first imaged outside yourself? Where has he or she been? Isn't it time to welcome him/her home? Isn't it time to know Asclepius as none other than the natural and wise essence of your heart and mind? Remain a few moments in this natural and noble essence. When you feel complete, slowly return to the time and place of the room, remembering that your ever-present inner healer will support and guide you toward integral health.

If I could offer a simple prayer for you, my readers, it would be this: May you be able to know the preciousness of your life, the beauty of your heart, and the qualities and capacities of your inner life. May you be able to use the well-endowed form of your body as a vessel to take you toward a life of meaning, depth, profound health, and service. May you begin with these preparations even if it takes a lifetime. As it is said in the East, "A bucket is not filled with water by the first or last drop. It is filled by the collection of a very large number of drops."

Psychospiritual Flourishing

We begin the shift toward integral health by first exploring the path to psychospiritual flourishing. We do so for four reasons. First, it is the most undeveloped aspect of our life. Second, it is a principal source of modern-day epidemics of mental suffering and premature disease. Third, it is the one area of our development that will most directly catalyze the full development of our life. Fourth, the development of our inner life is the most unique and precious opportunity given to us as humans. To forego its development is to ignore the final aim of human life—the opportunity to alleviate needless suffering and to gain health, happiness, and wholeness. For these reasons, it is essential to start with our inner life.

When we think of the mind, we usually think of the ceaseless mental chatter that occupies our days and visits us during the night as dreams. Beyond this, the mind is hard to describe. Ask someone to tell you something about his or her mind and the likelihood is you won't get much of an answer. Imagine if someone asked a similar question about our body. We would able to speak about organs, muscles, bones, limbs, cells, physiology, genetics, the probing images of MRIs and PET scanners, nutrition, fitness, and a great deal more. But when it comes to the mind—the author of much of our experience—there is little to say.

The West's exclusive preoccupation with the outer world has forced our inner life to go underground, and as a result, we have dismissed and devalued it. It has withered from lack of attention. As a result, we know less about the mind and how to use it than we do about our car or any household item. Although we may not be aware of this loss in our day-to-day life, it is what underlies the Western epidemics of our time. While it's unlikely we'll die from cholera, plague, typhoid fever, or other Third World diseases, it's highly likely that we'll suffer and die from Western epidemics of mental distress and stress-related degenerative diseases unless we undertake the unique opportunity for human flourishing.

The inner life of our mind, soul, and spirit has been an ongoing source of interest and exploration throughout history and across diverse cultures. But most often, this exploration has been an underground adventure undertaken by a few brilliant and hardy individuals who studied and practiced in isolation in the many mystery schools that survived in the shadows of culture. It is now time to move these mystery schools out of the dark and into the light.

THE FOUR LEVELS OF PSYCHOSPIRITUAL DEVELOPMENT

The famous Swiss psychologist C. G. Jung had a fascination with the inner life and those who sought to understand it. Among his varied interests were the alchemists, who spent 1,700 years trying to uncover the essence of the inner life. Of course they used the language of chemistry to do so, initially thinking they could find a way to transmute base elements into gold. With time it became apparent to them that the gold they were seeking through their symbolic approach was not physical gold but rather the gold that lies within. They were seeking the *lapis philosophorum,* the inner wisdom that could uncover the essence of human life.

Although they never created gold from dirt, they did outline with clarity and precision the complete path to psychospiritual flourishing. Forgotten and reduced to foolishness by others, Jung, in his unique brilliance, realized the richness of what they had left us—the contents of an intact mystery school elaborated in highly esoteric texts and images. In his extraordinary work on alchemy, he translated their work into modern terminology, mapping out the full evolution of our inner life. As a result, we are now able to understand this previously esoteric

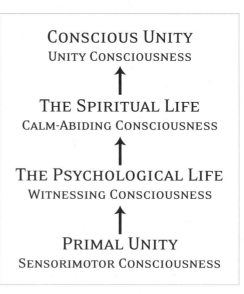

Figure 6. Psychospiritual Flourishing

process and to participate in the step-by-step evolution of our psychospiritual life from its most primitive form to its spiritual heights.

There are four steps to psychospiritual flourishing. Each step corresponds to a progressively more developed level of consciousness. Figure 6 shows each of these four levels in a way that expands upon Figure 2, allowing us to see how psychospiritual flourishing is inextricably related to the growth in consciousness.

We are born into a primal, *sensorimotor consciousness*. This is a very simple oneness and interconnectedness with life. For the infant there is no distinction between itself and the outer world. The newborn experiences through its senses and reacts instinctually with little or no consciousness. Remember that this is somewhat like poking the amoeba and observing its reflex reaction.

Early on, we lose this primal unity. This inevitable loss is necessary for further development because an unconsciously fused mind and body cannot evolve further. We are thus thrust into a psychological life with all its struggles, turmoil, reactivity, and isolation. Because Western culture does not, as a matter of routine, prioritize inner development at a young age, we are mistakenly forced to look outward to worldly experience as a way to calm our unconscious fears, insecurities, and losses that result from this broken oneness.

To successfully traverse this phase of psychological development, we must invest in our inner life by first becoming psychologically literate and healthy. The psychological process focuses on identifying destructive emotions and dysfunctional patterns and replacing them with a new set of healthy attitudes and behaviors. This requires the development of the next level of consciousness—*witnessing consciousness*. A witnessing consciousness allows us to stop, see, understand, and make choices about our thoughts and feelings. Intention substitutes for unconscious reactivity.

Once we have achieved a healthy psychology, it is time to leave the psychological focus and begin to explore the deeper nature of the mind. In this way, psychological development becomes a springboard for spiritual development. The spiritual process aims at penetrating the deeper layers of the mind to uncover the natural wisdom, inner peace, and loving-kindness that are the pivotal causes of a sustained well-being of body, mind, and spirit. This shift requires the development of the third level of consciousness—*calm-abiding consciousness*. Here, our faculty of intention matures. It becomes clear, focused, unbiased, and confident.

Through even further inner development, we develop the most subtle mind and reexperience the simplicity, oneness, and unity of the child. This final step requires the expansive and pure awareness of a *unity consciousness*. There is only one difference between this level of consciousness and primal consciousness, and it is a huge difference. This matured "innocence"—this very difficult and earned rebirth into a second oneness and simplicity—arrives with wisdom and consciousness. We now *know* our interconnectedness with all, and we can meaningfully use it help others and, further, to assist in creating a better world. It reminds us of the famous words of T. S. Eliot from his *Four Quartets:*

> *We shall never cease from exploration*
> *And the end of all our exploring*
> *Will be to arrive where we started*
> *And know the place for the first time.*

To know our inner home—to become fully aware of our true nature—is the nobility and glory of the human experience. Yet, in another sense, it is no more than the proper and normal unfolding of a fully lived human life. To progress through the levels of psychospiritual flourishing and achieve this full inner flourishing, we need a method. The method is contemplative practice.

CONTEMPLATIVE PRACTICE

The microscope and telescope are the tools we use to explore the outer world. Contemplative practice is the method and tool we use to explore the inner world and evolve our psychospiritual life. We use it in three ways. At first we use it to tame the mind's ceaseless mental activities that obscure higher states of awareness. Then, through mental training, we gain access to the more subtle levels of the mind—witnessing consciousness, the mental state of calm-abiding, and the pure awareness of a unity consciousness. The fully developed mind is a precise and sensitive instrument for inner inquiry, mind/body self-regulation, and the cultivation of the qualities of human flourishing—health, happiness, and wholeness. This three-step path to psychospiritual flourishing enables us to know and experience our mind and its multiple levels and capacities in the same detail that a microscope, MRI, or PET scanner allows us to know our body.

As medical science has gained understanding of the more subtle levels of the body—genetics and microbiology, for example—we have gained access to the more profound healing capacities of our biology. As a result, we have learned to work with our biology in a far more sophisticated way, expanding our ability to diagnose and treat illness. Similarly, as we gain access to the deeper levels of the mind through contemplative practice, we will discover previously unknown and unimagined inner resources and capacities. In both instances, expanding our knowledge of the inner and outer world takes us closer and closer to understanding and realizing our potential for integral health.

For example, in Chapter 2 we discussed the ability of the trained mind to influence our physiology, hormonal system, and immune system. We also noted recent studies suggesting that advanced contemplatives have gained the capacity to permanently enhance their well-being by altering the brain's neural circuitry. Brain research, called neuroscience, is now also exploring how contemplative practice can have a positive impact on attention, memory, perception, imagery, and a host of other mental functions. There is even some suggestion that much like working out a muscle, working out specific areas of the brain can result in structural change.

Research studies and personal reports have also demonstrated that mental training can transform the mind by reducing disturbing emotions that cause anger, hatred, fear, worry, confusion, and doubt while enhancing positive emotions such as patience, loving-kindness, openness, acceptance, and happiness. This mental transformation, acting through the mind/body connection, provides enhanced resistance to mental distress and physical disease, expands our healing capacities, and promotes well-being.

Yet there is more. An article written by Antoine Lutz and his colleagues at the University of Wisconsin and recently published in the *Proceedings of the National Academy of Science* compared contemplative scholars with a control group in order to study a particular kind of brain wave called the gamma wave. When the contemplatives were asked to develop a compassionate mental state, their brain waves showed a progressive increase and synchronization of gamma waves, which suggests a higher order of mental integration.

Currently no identifiable brain area or mechanism is known to bring together the activities of various aspects of the brain. It is just possible that what this study shows is the capacity of the trained mind to function at a higher level of integration and organization. These findings correlated with increased levels of clarity reported by the research subjects. And, further, the contemplatives had a higher level of synchronous gamma-wave activity when compared with controls even *before* the study began. This suggests that mental training may result in long-term changes as well as short-term ones.

There is another way to approach these mental Olympians without the use of machinery. We merely have to ask them what is happening in their daily experience. When we do that, we learn firsthand what machines may never be able to fully measure. They uniformly speak about the personal experience of well-being, universal loving-kindness, happiness, and wholeness unknown to the ordinary and untrained mind.

These self-reports document long-term sustained mental changes brought about through contemplative practices. Even the ordinary observer can see this by merely looking at their peaceful and joyful faces, feeling the warmth and embrace of their open hearts, and experiencing the contagious serenity of their presence. These testimonials and observations can be found throughout history and across diverse cultures and traditions. Such consistent reporting has a credibility all its own.

In a personal sense, contemplative practice offers us one more possibility. It offers us the opportunity to enter into a relationship with our inner self. It's not unusual for a beginner to blurt out, "I really didn't know there was anything inside me other than my thoughts and feelings." How would we know until we actually took a look inside! When we do, we find an entire universe within. I remember when I first began to discover this inner universe. It was a release and a profound refuge. It was as if a life-long burden had been lifted. The self I discovered was far different from the busy, striving, fearful, worrying self that had been my lifelong companion. Here was an aspect of myself that I could trust, that spoke the truth, that was content and at ease, that could surf life's adversities. No one could harm or take away this deeper self. It was an ever-growing fountain of peace, happiness, and wholeness. In short, I discovered an unknown source of a stable, profound well-being. These were not research findings. I knew them in my mind and heart.

As we undertake contemplative practice and explore the largely uncharted frontier of the mind, we will find a wealth of knowledge and capacity whose significance extends to our entire being. That knowledge impacts on our body, mind, and spirit. In this way, contemplative practice, which is the method that drives psychospiritual development, is actually an all-encompassing multidimensional integral practice. It is a way of "cross-training" our body, mind, and spirit all at the same time. It makes the most efficient and comprehensive use of our time. This is why psychospiritual development is a foundational aspect of integral health.

OUR MENTAL WORKOUT

We cannot earn a Ph.D. in physics without a daily commitment to study nor can an athlete attain an Olympian level of fitness without daily exercise. Similarly, it is not possible for us to evolve our psychospiritual life and access its capacities and resources without daily practice. Although the apex of human flourishing may require an Olympian intensity of effort and practice, we can be well on the road to health, happiness, and wholeness with a far more moderate yet sustained effort. One hour each day adds up, and it is not long before results can be seen. We know this from our own lives, from personal testimonies, and from research studies. We also know that like physical training, whether we are a pro or a novice, when we stop practicing, we will see a drop-off in our conditioning, whether physical or mental. So perseverance is necessary.

To gain the maximum benefit from contemplative practice, it is important to clearly understand the practices and methods that you will be using. For many years, I undertook practice without an understanding that went much beyond closing my eyes and relaxing. This may temporarily provide some ease and comfort but not much more. The most meaningful aim of contemplative practice is not rest and relaxation but rather the progressive development of an expanded consciousness and its healing capacities. An extensive catalogue of thousands of tested methods is available from the East where much of this work was pioneered. So we already have a track record we can count on.

In this book, we will address two types of contemplative practice. The first is *loving-kindness.* It opens our heart to others and gradually diminishes self-centeredness, priming our mind for further development. The second addresses the three levels of the subtle mind—witnessing, calm-abiding, and unity consciousness. It opens our mind and reveals a penetrating wisdom that knows the truth of our life and of existence. Loving-kindness and wisdom are the essential elements that heal at the source and drive human flourishing. Let's briefly explore them before we begin practicing.

Practice 1: Loving-kindness. The great sages have continuously reminded us that an enduring well-being requires a diminished focus on ourselves and our own needs and an enhanced concern and compassion for the welfare of others. Such a shift places us directly and firmly on the path to integral health and life. We already know from our own experience that loving-kindness attracts loving-kindness. We get back what we give. When we attract loving-kindness, our mind is calmer and a far better candidate for contemplative practice. Although, in the beginning, we must practice this mental attitude, there will come a time in the development of our psychospiritual life that loving-kindness will reveal itself as a natural and effortless aspect of higher consciousness. Then we will no longer have to cultivate this attitude or quality through practice.

Practice 2: The subtle mind. The wise ones also remind us that enduring well-being requires cultivation of wisdom. We cultivate wisdom by taming and training our mind, accessing its deeper levels, and exploring the essential nature of mind and experience. We begin by taming our busy mind. We learn how to diminish the ceaseless mental movements of thoughts, feelings, and images. If we practice regularly, we will definitely be able to still the mind and develop a witnessing consciousness that subsequently progresses toward the stable and facile mind of calm-abiding.

When stabilized, calm-abiding naturally evolves into the highest level of consciousness, unity consciousness. When we gain access to unity consciousness, we gain access to the resources of a higher consciousness—wisdom, peace, compassion, happiness, and wholeness. These capacities provide us with an extraordinary level and quality of insight and understanding that is not available to lesser levels of consciousness.

Together, these two practices help us to tame and train the mind, open the heart, expand consciousness, and progress us toward psychospiritual flourishing. They introduce us to the two wings of integral health—loving-kindness and wisdom.

⊠   ⊠   ⊠

A final word before we begin the practices. I have found from personal experience that in the beginning contemplative practice requires effort. But, let's face it, everything meaningful in life is achieved through effort, discipline, and perseverance. I assure you, however, also from personal experience, that once you undertake these practices, they will become such a source of peace and calm, ease and delight, creativity and wisdom that you won't want to stop practicing them. You won't want to leave your inner heaven. The initial problem, much like working out your body, will be sticking to your practice. But, at some point, the problem will be getting up from your practice and moving into your day-to-day life. Then, of course, as we will learn later in the book, the world must become your practice if you are to continue further on the path to human flourishing. So accept the diligence required to make the initial investment, and know that as time progresses, much like your physical workout—but even more so—you won't want to let go of contemplative practice.

GETTING STARTED

Traditional instructions tell us that it may be best at the beginning to do several short practice sessions of 5 to 15 minutes each day until you become more comfortable with longer periods of time. (This will diminish the number of problems you may encounter and encourage you to continue.) It is best to choose a certain time of day, preferably in the early morning, as your mind is most likely to be still before you begin your daily activities. Whatever you choose, you should place this time in your schedule as you would for other activities. If possible, it is helpful to set aside a place in your home that is private, comfortable, and conducive to silence. But you can always turn your gaze inward, even for a minute or two, to practice at any time of day and in any location. You will be amazed at how slowing the breath and turning your attention inward for even a few moments can make a considerable difference in how you feel and how you relate to others.

When practicing at home, some people prefer to sit on a chair, others on a cushion. The point is to be comfortable. Whatever you choose, be sure to hold a noble upright posture, opening your chest and heart and fixing your gaze a few feet in front of you with your eyes open or closed, as you wish. It's best to begin by feeling relaxed and at ease.

We are about to introduce the first practice of loving-kindness. I chose it as our first practice because it is important, easy, and gentle. It will ease your mind and open your heart, preparing you for the practices that follow. I recommend that you work with this practice for a week without reading further in this book. Giving this practice a full week will allow it to mature within you. It will also bring your experience of reading this book to life. It will become a living workshop and the beginning of an ongoing retreat. Setting aside time to practice rather than read will allow you to embody these words—to make them truly your own. It will also allow you to feel the changes that begin to occur and accrue as you establish your practice. It will not be long before you notice its effects on your well-being. So, for one week, devote your reading time to practice. That will also bring us closer together as we continue to grow through this book.

What I'm asking you to do is use this book as if it were a distant learning program or an online seminar that contains both text and specific assignments. But don't worry: no papers will be due; only your practice, direct experiences, and realizations. But like any teaching or training program, doing the homework—the practices—is essential. So try to focus your mind and organize your life as you would when undertaking any learning experience, setting aside time for both the reading and the practices. After six weeks, you will have completed the initial curriculum, started to gain the rewards, and be on the path to integral health and life.

Too often I have spoken at conferences only to discover that everyone goes home excited and motivated, but doesn't follow through, so nothing changes. At best, I was providing intellectual stimulation, at worst just entertainment. That is not what I wish for you. I wish you to use this book and its practices to bring integral health, happiness, and wholeness into your life. This requires focusing on the words in the text, reflecting on their meaning, and developing a certainty regarding their truth through regular practice.

I suggest you read through the loving-kindness practice once or twice before beginning. You have the option of recording it as a guided contemplation on an audiotape, jotting down a few notes to refer to while practicing, or remembering the basic content of the practice and proceeding without either of the above. Try different options to see what works best for you. Begin by identifying a 15-minute time period twice a day that will be inflexible for the week. (If you discover that fifteen minutes is too long at first, reduce your sessions as recommended above to 5 to 10 minutes each. When you are comfortable, you can increase the time to 15 minutes or longer.)

Locate a place that is both private and comfortable, in which you will not be interrupted. This is your sacred retreat space, so furnish it for this purpose. Place yourself in a comfortable position and have a timepiece nearby, *without an alarm,* which you can refer to as you reach the end of your 15-minute practice. Keep your eyes open or closed as you wish. If your eyes are open, fix your gaze a few feet in front of your body. Take a few deep breaths and relax into the natural peace of your body. Now you are ready to begin.

Practice 1: Loving-Kindness

Resting comfortably in your natural state of peace and ease, bring to mind an individual, someone close to you, who you hold with great love and tenderness. Allow these loving feelings to expand within your heart as if a faucet of loving-kindness were being fully turned on. Take a few moments to fully experience these feelings.

With these feelings filling your heart, begin to turn them toward yourself. Start with your body and its sensations, pleasant and unpleasant. Give each of them your love, your kindness, and a sense of ease, spaciousness, and care. You want to loosen any grasping or attachment to your sensations. Just let them be. Take a few moments to be at peace with your body and its sensations.

Next, shift to the thoughts, feelings, and images that move in and out of your awareness, those that are unpleasant and disturbing, as well as those that are pleasing and welcome. Give all of them equal care, love, and kindness, treating them as close friends that inhabit your life on a daily basis. Loosen any grasping or attachment to these mental movements. Give them a large field to play in.

Then, turn to your inner mind, specifically to the stillness, peace, and gentleness that is your natural home. Give this deeper aspect of your mind—your soul and spirit—all the loving-kindness that is in your heart. Welcome it into your life.

Finally, fully embrace yourself for the unique and precious expression of life that you are. Loving yourself is a prelude to extending this love out to others. Take a few moments to complete this part of the exercise.

Next, visualize a loved one who is now suffering. When you take your next breath, which we will call the "in-breath" from now on, take in your loved one's suffering. Allow this dark cloud of suffering to ride the in-breath into your body and then let it completely dissolve in your heart. Do not feel concerned about being overwhelmed by this suffering; its nature is such that it will dissolve if you merely breathe it into your heart. Then, when you breathe out, which we will call the "out-breath" from now on, breathe out health, happiness, and wholeness to the same loved one. Take in the suffering of your loved one on the in-breath, and on your out-breath send out health and joy. Continue this for several minutes. Consider how you can be of specific assistance to this loved one. What can you offer to relieve his or her suffering, temporarily and over the long term? Is it something material you can offer? Is it deep listening, understanding, a new perspective, emotional support? Or perhaps you can suggest a long-term strategy that will assist this loved one in identifying and eliminating the sources of distress. On your out-breath, offer what you sense will be most helpful.

Next, expand your focus to include a circle of strangers beyond your immediate loved ones. Breathe in their suffering and allow it to dissolve in your heart. With the out-breath, send out the peace and wellness that is growing within you. Continue this for several minutes.

Next, embrace all living beings, including those whom you consider enemies. Imagine this whole field of individuals is in front of you as you continue this practice of taking and giving.

Continue in this manner for the remainder of your practice session. Experience the changes that take place in your mind and heart. Remember this is an inner practice whose primary goal is to create a heartfelt loving-kindness that diminishes your self-centeredness and quiets your mind.

When the 15-minute practice time has passed, remain for a moment in the natural peace and ease of your mind and body, reflecting on the practice. If you wish, jot some notes in your journal. When you are ready, slowly and peacefully return to your regular activities. Continue this exercise twice daily for the first week and at regular intervals in the future.

With our preparations completed and our heart and mind softened by the loving-kindness practice, we are now ready to explore the further reaches of psychospiritual development. This next phase of psychospiritual development is very exciting as we become pioneers exploring uncharted territory. Each practice session brings greater skill and new insights. Our life becomes alive with the sprouting of new growth. We feel grateful and blessed, awakening to the possibility that we can actually change the course of our health and life. If we take on the practices with anticipation and perseverance, our initial faith will turn into confidence and then into certainty.

The Subtle Mind

7

We've reached toward the stars with spaceships and have mapped the physical universe, yet we have little understanding of our mind. As a result, we are unable to access its healing resources and life-enhancing qualities. However, through ongoing contemplative practice, we can train the mind, experience the subtle levels of psychospiritual development, and gain access to these resources and qualities. The undeveloped mind, which was once our greatest slayer, can then become our greatest healer. By attending to our inner experience, we begin to transform what is ordinary health into integral health.

Many metaphors can help us understand the mind. We can view the mind as an open and spacious sky. Or the mind can be seen as a vast and immeasurable ocean. Or it can be experienced as a clear and highly polished mirror. However, clouds can hide the spacious sky, waves can disturb the serene ocean, and images can obscure the clear mirror.

What these metaphors describe are *two* aspects of the mind: First, the ever-present still and clear mind—the cloudless sky, calm ocean, clear mirror—and second, the ever-changing moving mind—the clouds, waves, and images. The still and clear mind is usually obscured by the moving mind—the ceaseless mental activity of thoughts, feelings, and images. However, this subtle and still mind is essential for integral health and life. It is the source and storehouse of our most significant healing resources. To reveal it and access its resources, we must learn to quiet the seemingly uncontrollable and obscuring movements of our outer mind.

We can catch a peak at this inner essence in the silent space between two thoughts. Or we may experience it upon arising from sleep, in the brief moment before we are fully awake. Sometimes we get a glimpse when we are suddenly shocked by a sound, experience, or event that for a moment stops all mental activity. We can also experience it when we are immersed in the stillness of nature, which evokes the mind's innate stillness. If we are very observant, we will notice this same experience arises in the moments before and during sexual orgasm.

In these brief and evanescent moments, our mind is released from its preoccupation with mental chatter. It is at rest. Easily and usually missed, these moments are rare glimpses of the mind's subtle essence—its silence, spaciousness, peace, clarity, timelessness, and oneness with all of life. So if we look very closely, we will notice that the cessation of the moving mind allows the subtle mind to reveal itself. But most often, we simply enjoy the brief respite and the pleasurable feelings while the subtleties of this precious moment go unnoticed. Although we have a feeling that we have arrived home, we miss the real point. We've had the experience but missed its profound meaning.

We are far more familiar with the second aspect of the mind, the moving mind with its continuous stream of thoughts, feelings, and images. This stream of ongoing mental activity totally obscures the underlying essence of the mind. Yet it does not alter it any more than the clouds alter the vast sky. Contemplative practice aims at liberating our mind from its preoccupation with this endless chatter by teaching us how to tame and witness the moving mind rather than grasp and attach to it. With ongoing practice, we can then cultivate and stabilize the subtle mind. In this way, it becomes possible to access, sustain, and utilize the profound wisdom and healing resources that are innately present at this level of experience. Our brief glimpses can gradually become the center of our life.

There is a story about a merchant who visited a wise teacher. When he arrived, they started to talk. Shortly after, the teacher began to pour tea into the merchant's cup. He continued to pour the tea even as it overflowed the rim of the cup. The merchant shouted, "What are you doing?" The teacher replied, "The cup is like your mind. It is overflowing with mental activity, leaving no room for something new." Startled by the teacher's action and comment, the merchant's thinking process suddenly stopped and his mind became silent. Seeing this, the teacher said, "And that is the second aspect of your mind, its essence—the still mind." The teacher then began to speak to the still mind, relating the profound teachings that conveyed an understanding of the two aspects of the mind. So the teacher successfully used a startle technique to interrupt the moving mind, which allowed him to point out the mind's subtle essence.

As we pursue contemplative practice, we will progressively experience the three levels of the subtle mind: witnessing, calm-abiding, and unity consciousness. Our first step is to tame the mind and cultivate a witnessing consciousness. The second is to extend and sustain our mental control, achieving the still mind of calm-abiding. The third step is to stabilize calm-abiding as it gradually evolves into unity consciousness and pure awareness.

THE WITNESSING MIND

When we try to direct or focus the mind, it is not long before it is drawn back to our mental chatter. Our attention is continuously and involuntarily pulled toward this chatter. That is how the untrained mind works. With practice, we learn how to stop the mind's tendency to cling to random movements. Instead of grasping and ruminating, we learn to impartially observe and witness the natural rising and falling of thoughts, feelings, and images.

If we witness rather than grasp at random mental activity, it will naturally dissolve into the background from which it came. The mental activity that hides our deeper mind disappears. Our clear and still mind is revealed. This witnessing capacity is what we seek to develop first. If we can accomplish this, we gain a valuable piece of freedom. We will liberate ourselves from lifelong slavery to our mental movements, gain the capacity to choose where our attention goes, access our clear and still mind, and create the foundation for calm-abiding and integral health.

CALM-ABIDING

With practice and patience, the active mind is gradually tamed and subdued. It's transformed from its usual state of busyness to an increasingly sustained and effortless stillness. When the stillness is stable, we refer to this as the mind of *calm-abiding*. Calm-abiding is an unusual and remarkable accomplishment. The mind is undisturbed by the thoughts, feelings, and images that usually occupy our awareness. These mental movements simply arise and fall without drawing our attention or interest. We develop a "Teflon" mind. We abide in the stillness rather than in the turmoil of the mind's movements. It is like a great ocean unaffected by the rising and falling of waves.

What arises in this state is called mental and physical pliancy. No longer disturbed by its movements, our mind becomes light and soft. Intention replaces reactivity. Wisdom replaces confusion. Peace, serenity, and loving-kindness deepen our relationships and balance our physiology. We are now able to access the mind's deeper nature and its natural healing resources. In this way, we create the foundation for unity consciousness.

UNITY CONSCIOUSNESS

With this final level of psychospiritual flourishing, we can gain deep insight into ourselves and our life. The special wisdom of this subtlest mind sees directly, with the clarity of the inner eye, how things actually exist and work. As a result, our confusion, doubts, and misunderstandings dissolve, and needless mental distress and premature illness are healed at the source. We feel increasingly connected to all of life. We feel healthy and fully alive. We have finally gained the inner healing resources—the loving-kindness of an open heart and the wisdom of an open mind—that will take us toward sustained health, happiness, and wholeness.

Our ability to reliably access the deeper layers of the mind is what transforms a glimpse of what is possible into a way of life. Our intermittent glimpses provide an immediate experience, but they are transitory and undeveloped. As a result, we can neither sustain them nor can we gain access to the healing resources of consciousness. For this, we need to practice and progress through the levels of psychospiritual development.

With practice, we discover that there is a natural transition from witnessing consciousness to calm-abiding to unity consciousness. Each becomes the platform upon which the next level of development unfolds. As a result, we are able to progress through the psychospiritual levels of development with a single practice, *the subtle mind practice*. This practice teaches us to tame and stabilize the moving mind, develop a witnessing consciousness, shift into calm-abiding when possible, and experience unity consciousness when the earlier stages have been mastered.

There is a story told about an old Sufi who is walking through the forest late at night when he suddenly falls into an abyss. He quickly grasps a thick vine. For hours, he clings to it because the darkness prevents him from seeing the depth of the abyss. The evening turns cold and his hands begin to freeze. Moment by moment his grip loosens. Finally, filled with fear, he loses his grip and falls. But instead of falling into an abyss, he finds himself on solid ground. We do much the same. We cling for life to our active mind fearing we will be lost in an unknown emptiness. We cannot stay still. But when we stop grasping and leap into the unknown, we find that we are also standing on solid ground. Our fears were in vain. In fact, we are standing on the *ground of our being*. When we finally stop clinging to the movements of our mind, we discover that what we feared to be emptiness is actually our essence—a still mind and open heart that is free, at ease, and one with all existence. Witnessing and calm-abiding are preparation for this fall into our deepest self. That is unity consciousness.

PRACTICE 2: THE SUBTLE MIND

This practice will introduce you to the three levels of the subtle mind. It will become your basic daily practice, assisting you in progressing toward psychospiritual flourishing. You need to know that it will evolve over time as a daily practice.

We begin with a simple yet profound ancient practice related to the breath. We use the breath for two reasons. First, there is a direct relationship between the breath and the mind. You will notice early in practice that as your breathing becomes more easy and rhythmic, your mind will follow. Peaceful breathing pattern leads to a peaceful mind. Still the breath and you still the mind. Second, the breath is always with us so we can work with it even in the midst of a meeting. Using the breath, we will learn how to tame and stabilize the mind by developing a witnessing consciousness. As witnessing replaces grasping and clinging, we progressively experience calm-abiding, and calm-abiding gradually evolves into unity consciousness.

Before beginning this practice, review the instructions for the first practice in Chapter 6. Now substitute the following practice for the two daily periods you scheduled for the loving-kindness practice. However, I advise you to revisit the loving-kindness practice a few times a week. If you find it easy and comfortable, you may increase these sessions from 15 to 30 minutes. It will be best to review the instructions before each session until you're familiar with this practice.

Use the breath as a focal point. You can either focus on the rising and falling of your chest in the breathing cycle or the movement of the breath in and out of your nostrils with each inhalation and exhalation. Choose whichever works best for you. Begin by bringing your attention to your focal point. Start with ten deep in-breaths and out-breaths. Next, settle into the natural ease of your mind and body, breathing comfortably while maintaining firm concentration on your chosen focal point.

When thoughts, feelings, sensations, or images distract your attention, notice them and gently return your attention to the breath. It is like tying your mind to an immovable stake in the ground. In this case, the stake is your breath. Watch your mind carefully. If it escapes from the focus on your breath, bring it right back. This is a highly intentional, mindful, and to some extent even a forceful process. It is what is initially required to tame the busy mind. As the mind responds and its mental activity quiets down, gradually ease up on your grip on the breath. You will notice that you are now spending more time witnessing your mental activity and less time uncontrollably immersed in it. Pause here for several minutes and practice this focused concentration technique.

This is your opportunity to observe how the mind works. Watch its mental movements. Observe how you are involuntarily pulled toward random mental movements.

Can you see how your mind is trained to grasp and cling to them? What happens when you lose interest in and let go of mental movements? Where does the mental activity go? Can you see the difference in your mind and body between grasping and witnessing? Can you see how it is possible to transform the clinging and attaching mind to a witnessing mind? Can you see how a thought, feeling, or image naturally rises, abides, and dissolves if you leave it alone? Observe your mind and learn how it actually works.

Progress requires patience. Regardless of your efforts, you may lose your focus many times in each session. That's okay. Stay with the practice, and bring your attention back to the breath. Continue as long as necessary to settle and then explore your mind.

When your mind is less apt to grasp on to mental movements, slowly release the grip on your breath. You will still need to maintain your focus but with less force. It is like holding a piece of paper very tightly between your fingers and then slowly releasing your grip while still holding on. Your focus must be tight enough so that the mind does not get away and loose enough so that you are not tense. You will learn to cultivate this balance as you advance in practice.

There will come a time when your mind is firmly stabilized in stillness. This may occur in some sessions and not in others. When this occurs, you can slowly release your grip and shift your attention from the breathing cycle to the stillness itself. The stillness becomes your new focal point. This is a subtle and important shift. A small corner of your mind maintains attention on the mind's stillness, which is a far less tangible focal point. Now you can explore the still mind. What are its qualities? Does it feel contracted or spacious? Does it feel past or present? Does the stillness feel like relaxation or something deeper? Does it feel like the real you, like your true nature? Is this real you different from your usual sense of "I"? If so, where has your I gone? Is it merely another thought? If there is no I, what is left? Consider these important questions.

If your mind begins to wander, you must return to your breath until it resettles. Then you may ease up once again, shift your attention to the stillness, and abide in the stillness as you continue your inquiry. This will be a back-and-forth process that will change with each practice session. Continue this exercise, applying varying levels of effort as you practice taming your mind, witnessing its workings, and, finally, stabilizing it in calm-abiding.

When sustained, calm-abiding naturally evolves into unity consciousness. It is as if the spaciousness and stillness of calm-abiding expands and expands until it becomes all-encompassing. Then, unity consciousness and undisturbed awareness reveal themselves. Our deepest essence emerges. Our mind is clear, quiet, stable, open, alert, and all-knowing. Here, the mind drops into the heart. Separation, isolation, disturbing emotions, confusion, doubt, and an imbalanced physiology are healed by our innermost source. We have found our deepest nature and the natural healing resources of an open mind and an open heart.

Release your mind and allow it to float free. Experience everything with a clarity and vividness, but attach to nothing. Notice the quality of this choiceless awareness. What happens when you are aware without preference? Do thoughts, feelings, and images seem less real? Are they permanent or temporary? Where do they come from and where do they go? Do they belong to you or are they merely passing phenomena of consciousness? Is there a difference here between you and another individual? Is there intelligence in this pure awareness? Is it logical or intuitive? What is the difference between information and wisdom? Are there universal and unchanging truths? What is one of them? Is it possible that this level of consciousness may be the source of a constant and cultivated sense of health, happiness, and wholeness? Consider these questions.

Unity consciousness and pure awareness are the culmination of the subtle mind practice. This seemingly simple state of mind is a high level of attainment, so it will take time to achieve. Although at first access to unity consciousness may last only a few moments, our experience will grow with practice. Just the fact that we know that we can experience this innate natural home is quite important. We know that although we can forget it in the course of everyday life, we cannot lose it. For a few moments each day we can stop, look inward, and rest in this inner home. In this way, we will continuously train our mind to recenter itself in its innermost essence. Continue your practice until the end of the session.

When you are finished, slowly return to the time and space of the room, giving yourself a few moments to consider what you have learned. Perhaps you'll want to jot a few notes in a journal before you return to your routine activities.

NOTES FROM A FELLOW TRAVELER

Early on everybody asks, "What will I do if my mind won't quiet down?" The reality is that each practice session will be somewhat different. At times the mind may respond more easily than at others. When it just won't settle, you will have to be satisfied with observing how agitated your mind, body, and life actually are. The teachers tell us that in the beginning the mind seems like a waterfall, its noise becoming louder as a result of our going inward to observe it. Nothing has really changed except our attention to the mind. Then, with practice, the mind becomes like a rushing mountain stream, agitated but not as noisy as a waterfall. Gradually it becomes like a lazy river flowing through the flat plains, easy and quiet. In the final stages of practice, it becomes like a river reuniting with the still, deep, stable ocean. In any single practice session, you may go through each of these phases—the untamed mind, the increasing stillness of the witnessing mind, calm-abiding, and unity consciousness—or you may only encounter one.

It may also be valuable to observe the events of the day. Does the level of your mental activity during the day significantly affect your ability to stabilize your mind? Are all the telephone calls, conversations, and other distractions necessary? Are you perhaps too sleepy or exhausted before you begin your session? Can physical exercise or yoga help to stabilize your mind and prepare it for practice? Does the absence or presence of a recent meal affect your mind? Is the morning a better time for your practice or before eating or after exercise? You might also review your preparations. Have you adequately prepared your room to support your practice? Does your mind continuously return to a specific life problem? If so, you might stop, give this a moment of reflection, and then let it go and return to practice. If you carefully examine your experience, you will likely uncover the source of difficulties and come up with the proper remedy.

If you can find a skilled teacher to be your guide, you will be quite fortunate. Such a person can look in your eyes, listen to your experience, and help you with any problems. By "skilled teacher" I'm referring to an individual who has practiced and studied for many years within a tradition that aims toward inner freedom rather than mere relaxation. An increasing number of people and centers can serve this role. You will find several listed in the Resource Guide.

In this chapter, we have explored the three levels of consciousness—witnessing, calm-abiding, and unity consciousness. The practice I've described can assist you in exploring each of these levels. But this is a great deal of material. It is enough for a lifetime. In writing this book, I had to choose between giving you a simple, early practice that would serve more as a relaxation technique or exposing you to the full scope of psychospiritual flourishing. I have done the latter, knowing quite well that to bring these practices into your life and fully develop them will take you much time, preparation, effort, study, skilled teachers, and, of most importance, daily practice. To supplement our discussion and instructions and further refine your practice, I recommend *Genuine Happiness* by Alan Wallace. It is listed in the Resource Guide.

In the East, the lotus flower is the symbol of human flourishing. Its nascent bud represents this ever-present but undeveloped potential that lies unseen and unknown within each of us. Slowly, the growing bud makes its way through the mud, much as our human possibilities emerge progressively from the obscuring layers of an untrained mind and a closed heart. And once we have firmly turned toward our deepest self, gradually, petal by petal and realization by realization, our inner life will unfold. We will then be on the most direct path to a profound and enduring health, happiness, and wholeness.

Biological Flourishing

8

No one will dispute the importance of physical health as an essential component of integral health. The West has accomplished so much in the past 500
years that has enabled us to understand and assist the body in overcoming
many disabling and deadly conditions. We live longer than our ancestors did. We are
more capable of healing a variety of ailments, preventing others, and supporting with
dignity and care the inevitable process of disease, aging, and death. As we move into
the era of microbiology and genetics, there is still more to come. We must encourage
and support the ongoing efforts of modern science as it seeks to improve our health
and extend our life.

In the last twenty-five years, these efforts to improve physical health have gone
far beyond the diagnosis and treatment of disease. They now include a concern for
physical fitness, nutrition, preventive measures, and health promotion. However, these
important efforts expand but do not essentially change Western medicine's exclusive
focus on anatomy and physiology. As a result, we remain unaware of other aspects of
our biology, aspects that can only be discovered through an integral approach. That
approach requires us to move beyond a singular focus on the physical—beyond
anatomy, physiology, biochemistry, microbiology, and genetics—to the mental and
spiritual. Developing these aspects of our biology will help us evolve the full potential
of our biological life.

Figure 7 shows the major levels of biological development: anatomical, physiological, mind/body, and spiritual body. With each step up the developmental ladder,
we shift our focus and expand our horizon. This evolution toward a progressively
higher level of development, complexity, and capacity is essentially a movement from

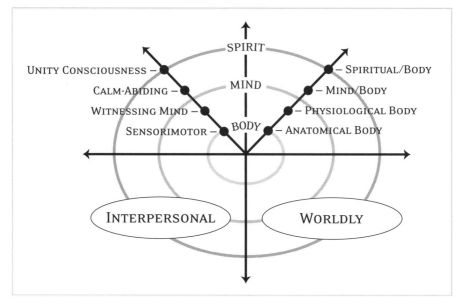

Figure 7. Biological Flourishing

body to mind to spirit—a process of development that applies to each of the four aspects of life. It is the generic pattern for the evolutionary unfolding of our human potential and integral health.

This developmental movement from body to mind to spirit is a shift in experience and identity from the realm of the physical with its emphasis on survival, instinct, and self to the more subtle and intangible realm of the mental with its focus on ideas, intention, and interconnectedness to the most subtle spiritual realm of awareness, wisdom, and oneness. This same development sequence is also a shift from *outer to inner to innermost*. Let's see how this fully unfolds as we move from the most physical levels of our biology—the anatomical and physiological—to the more subtle mind/body and spiritual body.

THE MIND/BODY

What do we mean by the mental and spiritual aspects of our biological life? The very question sounds like an oxymoron. But this reaction merely reflects a limited culturally learned understanding of our body that is linked to our narrow outer view. We have learned to approach our biology only through science. Science arrives at its understandings by reducing the body to its most physical elements. What we discover are the physical facts of our biology. But what happens if we approach biology from the perspective of our personal experience? What we then find is not a series of definable parts but the profound mystery of life that is encoded into our physical nature. We are now looking at the whole rather than the parts. From this perspective, our biology is no longer a problem to be solved but rather a mystery to be lived and explored first-hand. It is in this way that we discover the higher levels of our biology—the mind/body and the spiritual body.

We have already begun to grasp the bare essentials of a mind/body connection through our use of such techniques as biofeedback, practices of yoga and tai chi, and relaxation approaches. Our understanding has advanced further through research in the field of psychoneuroimmunology and the study of the capacities of highly trained contemplatives. We are now discovering that the body is a very sophisticated information system that is far more complex, ingenious, and dynamic than is suggested by a narrow anatomical view.

Our hardwired nervous system and our mobile messenger molecules manage the informational flow that goes from mind to body and back again. Together, these messenger systems keep the mind and body functioning as an interconnected whole. Understanding this allows us to use a variety of mind/body practices that enhance our well-being. Though we will still require a surgeon to remove a ruptured appendix, this expanded possibility offers us a new, more subtle level of control over our biology. We gain the capacity to shape our biology through mental training. Rather than ignoring the mind/body, let's use it.

How can we begin to shift our focus toward the mind/body? If even a small percentage of the resources spent on physical fitness were applied to mind/body activities, we would see a considerable gain in our society's general level of health. For example, let's look at our educational system. Perhaps school fitness programs could focus on mind/body fitness as well as physical fitness. Instead of just climbing ropes and doing calisthenics, we could add mind/body approaches like tai chi, qigong, or yoga to gym class. That way, we would be instilling in our children at a very young age a more expansive sense of their body and its relationship to the mind. Our children would aim to excel not only in physical fitness but also in mind/body fitness.

In addition to making cultural changes, we need to change our individual mindset. Close your eyes for a moment and imagine the interconnection of your mind and body. With the in-breath, breathe the mind into the body and experience it fully penetrating your cells, tissues, and organs. On the out-breath, breathe the body into the mind, allowing the body to fully penetrate your mind. Try this for five breathing cycles. Next, imagine information traveling between your brain and your body, between your kidneys and your heart, your foot and your arm, from your glands to your skin. Imagine a dynamic and interwoven movement of emotions, sensations, biochemistry, and physiology all moving together.

Now imagine that each aspect of your mind/body contains all the information and knowledge contained in all the other parts. You've just created a holographic mind/body. Which part of the pillow would you poke if you wished to make a change? Poke your emotions and you'll also be poking your hormones. Try shifting anger to loving-kindness and you will simultaneously shift your pulse, your skin temperature, and your immune system. Take a long hike in nature and observe the cascading series of changes in your entire mind/body. Notice how sensitive and responsive the entire system is to your mental attitudes and chosen environment.

So how do we translate this into daily life? Remember that physical workout we've become so accustomed to? We can now transform that into a mind/body workout. Try using your mind to enhance the results of your workout. Visualize the increase in strength, flexibility, and endurance you are developing through your workout. Let your mind assist you in achieving this goal. Many highly trained athletes use the mind/body connection as a routine part of their training.

Your workout offers another opportunity. Many fitness activities are repetitive and require little attention. So, while exercising, place your attention on your breath. Notice its movements. When your focus drifts, bring it back. When your mind is more still, shift your focus to the stillness. When distractions arise, allow them to naturally dissolve. When you are settled in stillness, allow your awareness to experience everything but attach to nothing. Continue this open, choiceless awareness. You may realize that you are now also using your physical exercise as mental training. Both are enhanced.

Isn't it true that our workout has never been totally about our body? Hasn't it also been about the ease and expansiveness that opens in our entire being? Isn't it true that we work out in part because it makes us feel more healthy, happy, and whole? These experiences are not a byproduct of physical activity alone. They also involve our mental state. If we approach our routine workout with this awareness, far more will be gained.

Much the same can be said for our contemplative workout. In actuality, these practices are not only mental and spiritual practices but also mind/body practices. As we still the mind, the body moves with it. Our breathing changes, our blood pressure and pulse are reduced, our muscles relax, our bowel motility diminishes, and so on. Is there a way to work out the mind and body separately from each other? That's impossible. So we're not creating something new; rather, we're recognizing what has always been. When we do that, we discover a whole new category of practices that can develop our mind/body system as a single unit.

This new type of cross-training involves mind/body activities such as yoga, tai chi, qigong, the martial arts, and other types of body and energy work. Here we actually work out the mind/body as a single unit. There is a fusion of physical movement and contemplative practice that brings us more in touch with mind/body interaction. We develop sensitivity to the subtle interconnection that has always been present though unnoticed.

How can this expanded focus help a difficult medical problem? Let's look at how we might apply an expanded vision of our biological life to pain. Pain may originate in our peripheral nerves, but our experience of pain takes place in the mind. If our brain was anesthetized, we would not experience pain. If we perceive pain as merely a physical phenomenon of the body, there is no other antidote than a physical one—be it a drug, surgery, or an acupuncture needle. All these may help and should be considered. But if we recognize that pain is a mind/body problem—a combined problem of our pain receptors and our mind—then it becomes possible to approach pain from a mind/body perspective and work with the mind as well as the body.

The experience of pain varies from individual to individual. This variation is largely due to the mental attitude of the individual. Fear and anxiety exacerbate the intensity of pain while mental training in a variety of relaxation techniques reduces the perception of pain. For example, breathing and relaxation practices help diminish the pain of childbirth and surgery, and biofeedback and visualization techniques reduce the pain associated with headaches and muscular tension. The same relief occurs when a soothing sense of reassurance and loving-kindness is conveyed from practitioner to patient. These are examples of how an understanding of the mind/body connection can extend our ability to work with significant medical problems.

Let's consider some other examples. We are all familiar with the ways in which out-of-control stress, negative emotions, rumination, and anxiety can impact on our body, affecting almost all of our bodily systems. Mental training does just the opposite. Biofeedback relies on amplified feedback from the body and mental training to control blood pressure, pulse, muscular tension, capillary blood flow, and bowel and bladder motility by reducing the hyperactive state of the body. This use of the mind/body can help alleviate migraine headaches, circulatory abnormalities, and gastrointestinal disorders. We also know that mental training can teach us how to shift blood flow in the brain affecting anxiety and depression and help enhance the effectiveness of the immune system. The doctor's perennial advice to "go home and calm down" reflects an astute view of the mind/body connection that has been gained through practical experience with ill patients.

Consider the number-one cause of death in our country—heart disease. We know from medical research that mental stress can cause an increase in blood pressure, pulse, heart arrhythmias, and diminished blood flow in already damaged coronary arteries. Each of these factors can accelerate the development of heart disease or slow recovery. We also know that an overly competitive, ambitious, and impatient attitude, called the Type A personality, can lead to a specific type of stress that is particularly damaging to the heart. Loneliness, depression, and social isolation are further risk factors for heart disease. Each of these is an example of the inextricable interconnection of mind and body. Even if you have an hereditary predisposition to heart disease, efforts to prevent its onset or aid in its recovery are greatly enhanced by mind/body approaches.

As we develop and integrate mind/body practices and therapies into our life and medicine, we will gradually gain a greater familiarity with this aspect of our biology. In time, we will begin to think in terms of the mind/body rather than body alone.

THE SPIRITUAL BODY

Like the Russian dolls enclosed within one another, we can access ever-deeper experiences of our body. The final stage in biological flourishing is the experience of our body as a manifestation of spirit. This leap is not easy for us in the West as we have been culturally steeped in the material solidity of the body, but it is quite simple and natural for those who have attained the further reaches of spiritual development. So for most of us, the following discussion may stretch our understanding.

It is simply not possible to fully know or reach the subtler levels of the mind/body or spiritual body without psychospiritual development. Though it is possible for any individual to have a sudden breakthrough that embraces all levels of biological development, it is unlikely that this will be a stable experience. Stability results from a gradual process of development. As we reach toward the higher levels of consciousness and progressively experience the more subtle aspects of the mind/body, we finally get a glimpse of the spiritual body.

A series of paintings by the contemporary artist Alex Grey entitled *The Sacred Mirrors* depicts what we mean by the spiritual body. As you stand in front of these life-size images, you see the movement from the solid anatomical body to the increasingly subtler levels of the body. The final image is of the most subtle body opening into and becoming one with all that is. Here we can see the full spectrum and interconnectedness of human biology as it moves from a solid anatomical body to a subtle mind/body to an immaterial spiritual body. Although we may not experience it as such, all are perpetually present at the same time.

Let's look at the immaterial spiritual body from a different direction. The study of subatomic physics shows us that our seemingly solid body is in fact more empty space than matter. Bones are made of minerals, minerals are made of molecules, molecules are made of electrons, neutrons, and other subatomic particles that move in the vastness of empty space. What we are learning from physics is that what appears solid is anything but solid.

Seen from yet another perspective, the physical stuff of our biology changes each day. The air I breathe today has visited each and every corner of the natural world, and the food I eat is a composite of elements that have taken many forms in the past and will be recycled again tomorrow. That's further proof our ever-changing body is not a solid body. Anatomical understanding of our biology is useful when a ruptured appendix needs to be removed, but it's very limiting when we seek to uncover our fullest human potential.

Those who have stretched the limits of the human experience offer us their view of the highest understanding of the body. The scholar John White has compiled various names given to this spiritual body. In the Judeo-Christian tradition, the spiritual body is called *the resurrection body*. St. Paul called it *the celestial body*. The Sufis call it *the most sacred body*. In Taoism, it is called *the diamond body*. In Tibetan Buddhism, it is called *the light body*. In Rosicrucianism, it is called *the diamond body of the temple of God*. In Tantrism and some schools of yoga, it is called *the vajra body, the adamantine body,* and *the divine body*. In Vedanta, it is called *the superconductive body*. In Kriya yoga, it is called *the body of bliss*. In Gnosticism and Neoplatonism, it is called *the radiant body*. In the alchemical tradition, the Emerald Tablet calls it the *Glory of the Whole Universe* and *the golden body*. In the Hermetic Corpus, it is called *the immortal body*. In ancient Egypt, it was called *the Akh*. In Old Persia, it was called *the indwelling divine potential*. In the Mithraic liturgy, it was called *the perfect body*. In the philosophy of Sri Aurobindo, it is called *the Divine Body*. In the philosophy of Teilhard de Chardin, it is called *the ultrahuman*.

Most of us would describe the many capacities or qualities attributed to the spiritual body as miracles. We are told about unexplainable healings and of "physical" accomplishments that are unimaginable given ordinary consciousness and our usual solid sense of the body. We've heard stories about extended survival, weightlessness, the ability to be in more than one location at the same time, extrasensory capacities, luminous bodies, super-vitality and movement, intuitive experience, transcendence, transformation, resurrection, and mystical ecstasy. When we consider these exceptional extensions of our biology, we are relying on personal testimonies. And yet, in some unknown way, these testimonies touch something in each of us that senses human beings are far more capable than we have been led to believe. So whether or not we take these literally, they point us in the direction of extraordinary human possibilities.

When there is even the slightest sense that our personality, body, and ideas about life and death are not as solid as we once thought, we have opened the door for the possibility of a certain type of immortality. In so doing, we have begun to soften the great existential fear of aging, disease, and death. By diminishing this fear, we experience a simultaneous release of many related fears of insecurity, lack of control, isolation, and separateness. These are replaced by previously unimagined ease and comfort. We surrender to life and we surrender to death. In doing so, disease and death as we ordinarily know them paradoxically come to an end.

Although it is highly unlikely that any of us will attain the levels of development described by the great mystics, we can gain a great deal by understanding the full spectrum of biological flourishing. When we are freed from the prison of an exclusively anatomical perspective, we attain the capacity to control aspects of our anatomy, biochemistry, physiology, microbiology, and perhaps even our genetic structure. When we attain an even more subtle experience of our biology, we simultaneously gain the possibility of extended human abilities as well as a liberating understanding of the true nature of disease and death.

But there is more. As we move from a fixation on our anatomy to subtler understandings of our biology, we begin to break through the sense of a solid and separate self. Higher consciousness opens further realms of our biology that a reductive science cannot know. Our span is greater as we perceive the interconnection and interpenetration of mind, body, and spirit. An ease and lightness enter our life and cleanse our mind and body. In this manner, biological development progressively extends our ability to prevent mental distress and physical illness, enhances recovery from disease, and promotes integral health, happiness, and wholeness. This is the gift of the full spectrum of biological flourishing.

Interpersonal Flourishing

9

We began our journey to integral health by focusing on the development of the psychospiritual and biological aspects of life. Yet we do not live in isolation. We live in relationship to others who are a bridge between our inner and outer life. Relationships, the third aspect of our experience, can be a living laboratory for interpersonal and psychospiritual development. They challenge us, teach us, and if we fail to learn their lessons, they teach us again. If we know how to transform them into potent practices, as we will discuss in this chapter, they can become an essential part of our path to health, happiness, and wholeness.

RELATIONSHIPS, HEALTH, AND HUMAN FLOURISHING

We can feel the impact of relationships on our health. We know what happens to our body when we are dissatisfied and struggling in our relationships. That is in sharp contrast to the feeling of lightness and ease that occurs when our heart is open and we feel the mutuality of loving-kindness and support. There is no doubt that the growth in our capacity for relationship—the movement from a focus on self to others— enhances our well-being. Decades of research confirm our personal experience.

Consider the following research that shows that healthy relationships of all sorts are a buffer against the effects of mind/body stress. In 1983, W. Eugene Broadhead of the University of North Carolina School of Public Health published an article in the *American Journal of Epidemiology* that reviewed a decade of research linking disease and premature death rates to the absence of supportive relationships. That study showed the protective effects of relationships extended to a variety of chronic and infectious diseases, pregnancy outcome, psychological illness, and suicide. Relationships were also shown to have a positive effect on recovery from illness and chronic disease. These effects have been verified again and again by large cross-cultural studies.

But do relationships have a positive effect on health beyond their impact on disease and recovery from illness? Here we run into a problem. Western medicine has been exclusively focused on disease rather than health. Many studies define the factors that lead to premature disease and death, but few if any scientific studies explore the factors that lead to authentic health and well-being, let alone human flourishing. For this, we have to extrapolate from the studies such as that noted above and rely on our intuition, personal testimonials, and the emerging research on contemplative scholars who are skilled practitioners of loving-kindness and exemplify good heartedness. Each of these sources of information points us in the same direction. The extent to which we can develop and reach out to others with intimacy, loving-kindness, and compassion will help determine how far we travel down the road to integral health and human flourishing.

THE CHALLENGE OF INTERPERSONAL RELATIONSHIPS

Dealing with relationships poses challenges on many levels. Once I attended a lecture given by one of the world's foremost teachers of human flourishing. He was teaching about loving-kindness and compassion. Sitting directly in front of me was a rather difficult person who was constantly moving about and disturbing everyone in a very crowded area. I could feel anger and irritation rising within me. So my ears were listening to a talk about loving-kindness and compassion, and my mind and body were thinking and experiencing anger. At that moment, where was the actual teaching? Was it coming from the teacher or from the real life experience with the person right in front of me?

It was easy to hear and feel the wise words, but it was far more difficult to deal with my built-in self-protective reactions to this individual. So, at that moment, my real teacher—my real life challenge—was sitting right next to me. Could I witness my anger rather than react to it with my mind and body? Could I maintain an inner calm regardless of my tendency to react? Could I practice patience, understanding, loving-kindness, and compassion in this situation? Could I feel the suffering of this other person? It is unimaginable that I might even be grateful to this individual for the lessons she was teaching me through her actions? Could I walk my talk? If not, what did all the lovely words mean?

This outer confrontation forced a confrontation with my inner life. How would it feel if I had spent many years practicing loving-kindness only to find my anger uncontrollably rising when I was confronted with an unpleasant circumstance? I had to grow inside or suffocate from my own anger. That is an example of how an interpersonal relationship can challenge us to further evolve our life, use our daily experiences as practices, and in this way progress on the path to integral health.

The poet Rainer Maria Rilke speaks to the challenge and opportunity of relationships with the following words:

> For one human being to love another human being: that is perhaps the most difficult task given to us, the ultimate, the final problem and proof, the work for which all other work is mere preparation. . . . Love does not at first mean merging, surrendering, and uniting with another person. . . . Rather, it is a high inducement for the individual to ripen, to become something in himself, to become world, to become world in himself for another's sake. . . .

With commitment, effort, and proper guidance our relationships *can* evolve and flourish. They can be transformed from an initial preoccupation with ourselves and our needs to an increasing concern for the other and their needs to a universal loving-kindness and finally to a sense of oneness with all. We grow from ego-centered dependent relationships to genuine intimacy to spiritual interconnectedness—from I to you to us to all of us. If we take up the challenge of relationship, it will take us toward interpersonal flourishing and integral health.

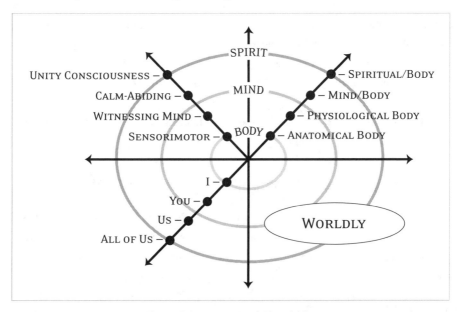

Figure 8. Interpersonal Flourishing

DEPENDENT RELATIONSHIPS

We cannot love others until we love and care for ourselves. This is a particularly vexing problem in the West where our inner life has been devalued and denied from childhood on. A parent without an inner life grows a child without an inner life. A parent without an inner connection grows a child without an inner connection. As a result, most of us have never touched our deepest essence—all that is good and beautiful within. So we learn to look toward others to find what we don't know is really in ourselves.

So we reach outside of ourselves for the comfort, security, and happiness that was lost with our forsaken inner life. We cling to others to satisfy our emotional needs, and we dress this up in nice words and call it love. In truth, we have a relationship with our own needs rather than a meaningful relationship with another. Pleasures derived from such relationships are like candles that invariably burn themselves out one after another. Without a genuine inner life, authentic intimacy with another is not possible. We cannot find outside what we must first find inside. So we are left with confusion, disillusionment, and suffering in contrast to the growing health, happiness, and wholeness that arise from more evolved relationships.

We can measure the degree to which our current relationships are contaminated by dependency by assessing the extent of our attachment to them. Would losing them leave us feeling empty, without any resources for peace and wholeness? To what extent do we give up the authenticity of our own lives for another? Are our most personal relationships filled with strife and suffering or permeated with joy? Relationships contaminated with attachment and dependency keeps us stuck and suffering rather than growing and flourishing.

Psychospiritual development will help us transform dependent relationships. With proper guidance, inner inquiry, and contemplative practice, we can gain needed insights, learn to freely open our heart, and reconnect with our inner home. Then we will be able to meet others in intimacy rather than need.

INTIMACY AND SPIRITUAL UNION

The shift from dependent relationships to intimacy is most often driven by exasperation, suffering, and an authentic desire to connect with others. Dependent relationships force us to see things about ourselves that we would prefer not to see. If we can accept this as a gift rather than as a curse and embrace a process of self-exploration, new insights will burst forth, the tight focus on ourselves will soften, and we will slowly develop a more expansive and rewarding concern for others. This will create the basis for authentic partnerships and genuine intimacy. It is then possible to care for another with empathy, communicate with honesty, love without judgments, and explore the profound depths of sexual union.

I'd like to share a personal experience that can demonstrate how a relationship can drive growth and development. Many years ago I shared an important relationship with a very special individual. Throughout our relationship, she repetitively asked me the following two questions: "Why can't you see me as separate from yourself?" and "Why can't you meet me?" For years I was confused by these questions, which frustrated both of us, led to much distress, and stopped the further development of our relationship. Only after my inner life began to develop was I able to understand the meaning of these questions. How could I see her if I was completely absorbed in my self, in my needs, in my fears, in my own mental activity? Everything she said was interpreted through the filters of these emotions. In actuality, I had a relationship with myself, not with her.

To move beyond this meant that I first needed to develop an inner witness. Then I could first see how my self-absorption denied me any opportunity to know my partner separate from myself. Next, I had to develop a still mind so I could actually listen to and hear her without interpreting, judging, or coloring what was being said. Only then could I know her as a unique person. Only then could she feel heard, seen, and known as an individual separate from my inner experience. Only then was intimacy possible.

The second question—"Why can't you meet me?"—was even more confusing at the time. In time I learned that love and connection cannot flow across a closed heart. Protectiveness, defensiveness, self-righteousness, self-absorption, judgment, interpretation, and all those other ways we have learned to cover over the vulnerabilities of childhood close the heart, shutting it tight. But intimate connection requires the heart. It requires listening to and knowing the other for whom they are. It means acknowledgment and acceptance. It means feeling the other almost as oneself. This was what she meant by "meeting her." To meet another, I discovered, was about the heart meeting the heart. She was asking for true intimacy.

It takes time and effort to master the skills that support authentic intimacy. Few of us acquire them from our families, and we don't learn them at school. So it is of little surprise that we have difficulties until we consciously undertake the effort to become "intimacy literate." This choice is not simply a choice about relationships. It is a choice to step out of the preoccupation with ourselves and increasingly value and care for another. It is a choice that places us on the path to integral health.

As we gain the capacity for intimacy and practice it in daily life, it slowly becomes possible to go further. It becomes possible to experience the deepest aspect of intimacy—a spiritual union. Such a union is not one of personality meeting personality but rather of presence meeting presence, life meeting life, divinity meeting divinity. This sacred union of two is a spiritual communion.

Practicing Intimacy and Spiritual Union

You and your partner may share the following practice. Allow an hour in a peaceful environment. Review the practice together several times before you begin.

When you are both ready, begin by sitting face-to-face and knee-to-knee. Take the first 20 minutes to individually, with eyes closed, follow practice 2, the subtle mind practice in Chapter 7.

After 20 minutes have passed, open your eyes and look directly into each other's eyes while maintaining your inner silence. The other's essence will now become your focal point. If you become distracted, resettle your mind and then bring it back to this focal point, allowing any thoughts, feelings, or inner images to dissolve. Stabilize your mind while looking deep within your partner.

You are now looking through your partner's eyes into the stillness of his or her soul. Remaining in silence, experience the vast presence beyond words. Feel the connection that goes beyond the known. Recognize the oneness and timelessness present in the other as it is in yourself. If mental movements arise, do not grasp at them. Let them dissolve. Then return to a stable, clear, and calm mind. Experience this union. Continue for another 20 minutes.

Become aware of how profound your understanding, insight, and connection can be. You are meeting your partner heart-to-heart and soul-to-soul. Here we are in intimacy and union with the divine in the other. That is true union. It is both personal and impersonal at the same time.

Gather the love from your heart and allow it to meet with the love from your partner. This love can then expand into the vast open space of pure awareness and spiral out to the universe. When two are united in this manner, they dissolve into a third—the wholeness and unity of life. Embrace the fullness of the universal heart. There is no clinging, no attachment, no you and no I. There just *is*. Remain in silence and communion for the final 20 minutes of your session. When you have completed the exercise share your experience with your partner.

There will come a time when you will reflect with wonder and awe on the distance your relationship can travel—from dependency to intimacy to spiritual union. This is the distance traveled from a closed heart and mind to an open one—from limitation to flourishing. It is the path to integral health.

UNIVERSAL LOVING-KINDNESS

It may appear at first glance that what we have discussed here applies only to intimate romantic relationships. But that is not so. As our consciousness expands, so does our reach. Our capacity for empathic listening, seeing, and caring for the other—open heartedness, sensitivity, generosity, and emotional intimacy—can spread to all our relationships. To see another, acknowledge another, hear another, be present with another, and feel one with another—a lover, a partner, a friend, a stranger, and even an enemy—is a profound healing gift for oneself and the world. Integral health requires that we begin to extend these capacities beyond our close group of loved ones to all of humankind. The development of universal loving-kindness is the final leap in our interpersonal development.

Try the following practice. Close your eyes and for a minute or two rest into the natural ease of your mind and body, and repeat the following phrases for 10 minutes.

> *May all individuals gain freedom from suffering.*
> *May all individuals find sustained health, happiness, and wholeness.*
> *May I assist all individuals in gaining freedom from suffering.*
> *May I assist all individuals in finding health, happiness, and wholeness.*

This mini-practice can be quite powerful in expanding your mind and heart. It can serve as an antidote to anger and hatred. It can help to shift your focus from personal love to universal loving-kindness. You can work with it at any time.

ONENESS

Separateness is an expression of cultural conditioning. It is not a deeper truth. We discover this only as we move beyond the limitations of lesser levels of consciousness through daily contemplative practice. We discover that we have two experiences: a sense of separateness that arises from an undeveloped consciousness and a sense of oneness that arises from a more subtle consciousness. Which should we believe?

The answer is that they are both valid experiences. So perhaps the better question is: Which do we choose to have as the center of our experience? If we choose the former—the experience of our uncontrolled personality—we will live in a world of separation. Such a life will be a roller coaster of pleasure and suffering. Integral health will remain illusive. If we choose to live from a sense of oneness—the experience of a higher consciousness—we will gradually learn to identify ourselves with the interconnection and interdependence of life rather than the narrowness of our personality. When we experience this sense of oneness with others, we discover that to give to another is to give to ourselves, to heal another is to heal ourselves, to be in union with another is to be in union with all. And this brings us toward integral health, happiness, and wholeness.

NOTES FROM A FELLOW TRAVELER

Close your eyes for a moment and create an image of yourself. Observe your separateness. Pause for a moment. Now add the image of an important individual in your life and reach out with intimacy and care. Observe the feeling of connection. Pause again. Now bring to your field of awareness all of your friends and family. Again, reach out to them with loving-kindness, support, and devotion. Observe how it feels to be open and to give to others. Pause once more. Finally, bring to awareness the presence of all humankind—all races, religions, and cultures. This field of awareness will extend out indefinitely. Open your arms and heart to all. Take in suffering and give out health and joy. Allow yourself to dissolve into a single universal heart. Observe how this universal and interconnected embrace feels. Pause for several minutes before you return to the time and space of the room. Consider this movement from I to you to us to all of us. Remember this brief practice and work with it again.

Perhaps nothing is as rewarding as the embrace of others. All healing traditions speak of this power of the open heart. We all know from personal experience how it feels to fully love and be loved. Yet too often the love we give and receive is more about ourselves than about others. We fear so we cannot be vulnerable. We protect ourselves so we cannot be fully open. We need control so we cannot surrender. We crave attention so we cannot be devotional. But as we expand our consciousness, we soften these barriers and our heart and arms slowly open. We discover that we get love by giving love and that love is abundant rather than scarce. We flourish in our relationships.

Flourishing in the World

10

Our day-to-day participation in the outer world extends from our individual relationships to our family, local community, nation, and planet—from small family dinners to global institutions. To flourish in the outer world means that we evolve our worldly life as we've evolved other aspects of our life. Expanded consciousness and matured relationships are the foundation for a meaningful outer life. Together, they assure that our physical health will flourish rather than suffer. Each is essential for a comprehensive and far-reaching integral well-being.

There is much we could cover here, but I think it is best to focus on our most immediate relationship with the outer world—our relationship to work. The experience we gain growing and developing this relationship can be a model for all our otherworldly endeavors—from an anonymous phone conversation to complex day-to-day involvement with political, social, environmental, educational, and medical institutions. The process is the same. Step-by-step we expand the awareness and consciousness we bring to our worldly experiences. In this way, we take what is seen as mundane and infuse it with a higher meaning and purpose. We spiritualize our worldly life, transforming ordinary activities into sacred ones.

OUR WORK IN THE WORLD

The term "our work in the world" has a double meaning. The first refers to the usual way that we view our work as a mere matter of necessity, as something we do to survive. The second view sees work as an opportunity to serve. From this perspective, work is a calling, a way to serve others regardless of the nature of our work. Flourishing in our work is to transform the first, work as survival, into the second, work as service. We need to take several steps to move from one to the other: from work as survival to work as creative expression to work as fulfillment of our longing for health, happiness, and wholeness, and finally to work as service.

However, the glaring reality is that our culture doesn't recognize work as service. Our cultural preoccupation with the economics of work ignores our inner life and then drives it underground. Our soul and spirit have no place at the worksite. We have become so accustomed to and disheartened by this reality that many of us have lost hope that there is something more than simply receiving a paycheck. We no longer feel we can find consistent meaning and fulfillment in this aspect of our life. We settle for survival. As a result, as we discussed in Chapter 2, worksite stress is a major cause of mental distress and premature disease—a fact that is now well documented by research and accepted by occupational health specialists and corporate leadership. However, work doesn't need to be a path to ill-health. It can also be a path to integral health.

If we seek more, we must ask how our work can take on meaning and purpose. How can it best serve our growth and development? This is different from seeking the perfect job or a perfect world. Of course we should look and hope for work that is best suited to our needs, capacities, and aspiration, but what we are seeking on the integral path is how to create something more out of what we already have, how to turn all of our experiences into practices. If we can learn this, then we can transform even the most difficult outer situation into an opportunity that will enhance our well-being and promote integral health.

Figure 9 outlines the four levels of development, which we will explore by using work as an example. At its most basic level, work can be nothing more than finding food and shelter, an act of survival and security. But it does not need to stop there. As we grow, our inner work can become an opportunity for creative expression, meaning, and fulfillment. With a further leap in consciousness, we can discover and experience our work as spirit-in-action, as engaged spirituality whose aim is to serve others with loving-kindness and care.

TRANSFORMING WORK

For many of us such a transformation may seem more like a dream than an actual possibility. We feel we have little choice when it comes to work. We see few, if any, options. We feel compelled to work out of financial necessity and the desire for job security. We are subject to the wishes of our supervisor or the needs of our corporation and its profit line. We don't feel in control of our work, and at times we may even

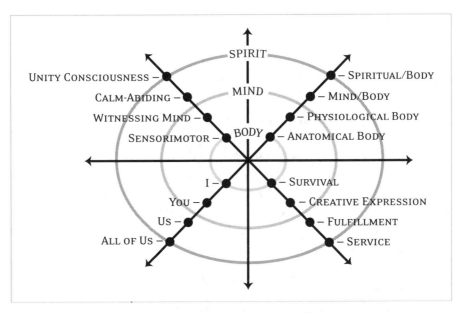

Figure 9. Flourishing in the World

feel victimized. This can set up a cycle of resentment, anger, and stress that is then reflected in our effectiveness at work and in mental distress, mind/body disturbances, and degenerative diseases. So how do we deal with these realities? How do we grow and transform this circumstance? How do we overcome this seeming obstacle to integral development?

Let's again turn to the great healers, listen to their advice, and find a way to translate their wisdom into the realities of our contemporary work life. The advice they give is quite simple and yet at the same time very difficult to accomplish for it is an *entire* integral path in itself. Although our path will be far more gradual, I am not going to dilute the pure essence and truth of their advice. The great teachers tell us to commit ourselves fully to our work without any regard for personal gain or loss. Regardless of the nature of your work, they say to let go of your usual outer self with its ambitions, striving, and judgments and focus only on the service and good you provide to others. Surrender your smaller self. Let your ego die in your work. Cease looking for what is right for you and ask how you can serve others. The sages say that selfless service to others is the quickest way to transform your work. If you can do this naturally, completely, and immediately, you can then flourish in the world irrespective of what is placed in front of you.

However, this is not a leap we can make all at once. It is a view from the mountaintop. First we must cultivate the lower fields. It is a process of progressively grow-ing our inner life and then allowing our expanding awareness to spill into our outer life. In this way, the shift will occur with naturalness and ease. We begin with small steps that slowly evolve our relationship to work in the here and now.

Beginning with Small Steps

Consider the following. For many years I have worked with physicians and other heal-ers who are disturbed by the lack of personal relationships with their patients. They no longer experience a heart connection or a sense of the soul and spirit in their work. They experience medical practice as an empty chore. Many reasons explain this. Fore-most are the many life-denying aspects of our current medical-care system. Yet I always remind my fellow practitioners that the moment they close their office door, the moment they are face-to-face with another individual, there is always a precious opportunity for open-heartedness, loving-kindness, empathic listening, and presence. This is the moment for their soul and spirit to flourish.

In that moment of direct contact, there is always the possibility of an intimate human connection, regardless of obstructive outer circumstances. If we open to this human connection, value it, and consciously try to live it, these few moments are worth far more than an hour spent exchanging information. To those physicians who feel they are too busy, I suggest they stay late one night a week or leave a couple of hours open one day each week to sit with a single patient as long as it takes to fully lis-ten and tend to the other in a spirit of communion and care. What I am suggesting is that healers take this time to practice their work as service, bringing to it their highest wisdom, loving-kindness, compassion, and integrity. I ask them to spiritualize their work at least once a week and experience what comes back to them from this shift in intention.

Anyone in any job or profession can take this first step. Try taking one of your many daily personal contacts and infuse it with kindness and care. This merely requires a choice, a presence, and an open heart. Then see what happens to you, to your heart, soul, and spirit. I think you will agree this is a small but potentially important step in finding meaningfulness and fulfillment in work.

Here is another suggestion. During a lunch break, stop and allow your breath to take you inward to a calm inner state. Relax into the ease of your body and mind. Let your work and your mental activity dissolve into your deeper awareness. Try this for just a few minutes at other times of the day. Just notice in the moments following this whether anything has changed in your work experience and in your sense of well-being. The mind returns quickly to its old ways so become an astute observer. If you know just once that you can change your experience of work by shifting your inner life, then it only takes time and practice until you can stabilize this inner and outer shift. You can be assured that not only will your work change but your coworkers will also change.

Here's another way to look at work. All work, whether it is the construction of a house or a road, sales or marketing, plumbing or police work, has at its core service to others. All work is a cooperative venture that supports each of us. Writing at my computer requires support from the woodcutter, mill worker, carpenter, and construction team that built the cottage where I live and the furniture on which my computer rests. Then there is the plumber and electrician who made this cottage livable, the farmer and store owner who provide the food that sustains me, and let's not forget the computer people who created the machine I write on and the people who taught me how to type. All these individuals are part of the book you are reading, including yourself.

If we continue this line of reasoning, we will soon realize that our current life is sustained through the efforts of many people. Although the ultimate impact of your work on another's life cannot always be seen at first glance, it is there. Each contribution is an essential piece of the whole. Without this interdependence and cooperation, none of us could meet our daily needs in the complex society we live in. Consider the role of a single neuron in the brain. It does not realize that it is part of a complex web of brain cells that together create an integrated mental activity. Although it cannot see its part in the whole, without it nothing would happen.

Close your eyes for a few moments and consider the links that connect us to one another. Consider how your work might have meaning for others, how it might serve others, how it is part of the larger whole. Can you see how your efforts are essential and irreplaceable, without which things would fall apart? Can you see this purpose and connection in all you do? Unlike the single neuron, we can comprehend our relationship to the whole. If you do so, this will be another way to find authentic meaning and purpose in your work.

Finally, try viewing all that you do in a larger context. When you are doing household chores, you can say to yourself that you are purifying your body and mind. When you are opening a door, it is opening the door to an integral life. When you are cutting the grass, you are cutting away the inner obstacles to that life. When you are listening to another, you are hearing everyone. When you are speaking, imagine precious gems coming from your mouth. When you are driving, imagine you are coming closer to your destination of health, happiness, and wholeness. Every aspect of your work can be a teaching and a practice, regardless of the kind of work you do.

If we continue our inner practices and try these and other small experiments at work, an unexpected miracle will begin to occur. We will see an alchemical transformation that turns dirt into gold. Nothing that we can see with our senses changes, yet everything begins to change from the inside out. What was once merely an effort at survival can slowly, through our own efforts, become a source of creative expression, meaning, and fulfillment.

Learning from a Woodcarver and a Psychologist

A story is told in the East about a woodcarver who was commanded by his king to create a bell stand. The woodcarver didn't have much choice. Perhaps he had other plans, in which case he could have become angry and resentful, feeling victimized by the king's demand. But that was not the course he chose. The woodcarver accepted what was required and began preparing himself. He fasted for three days and then intensified his contemplative practices, taming his mind so that it was completely emptied of negative emotions, of ambition, greed, pride, and any thought of the king.

When he was finally ready, the woodcarver skillfully brought his mind to stillness, and with complete focus on *his* work, he went into the forest, saw the bell stand already completed in the perfect tree, and then cut away the excess wood. The king was amazed at the beauty of his creation and could not understand how he had done it. "Was it the work of the spirits?" he asked. No, it was the work of a wise master.

The woodcutter had transformed the king's demand into an act of personal choice, discipline, and reverence. An outer order became, through the alchemy of his wisdom, an inner opportunity to engage his mind, heart, and spirit in the perfection of his work and life. He spiritualized the entire process, transforming a simple demand into a great treasure. This is the miracle of transformation. Do not think this inner miracle, this inner wisdom and skillfulness, is only possible for a mythical woodcarver. It is also in you. It is in everything you touch, even though you may not yet have the vision needed to see the hidden gold.

If we can accept our destiny, we can then embrace it, shape it, and make it our own. We can gracefully and wisely mine the possibilities present in what is given to or asked of us. In this way, we flourish in our world, not because our world is perfect, but because we bring beauty and spirit to it. We perfect the world through the force of our own inner perfection.

What better example can we have but the life of Viktor E. Frankl. Frankl relates in his book *Man's Search for Meaning* how he infused purpose and spirit into his unchosen life in a concentration camp. He tells us that those who could not find meaning, even in this most dire circumstance, were the quickest to die. He survived, flourished, and went on to develop a form of psychotherapy called logotherapy. We are again reminded through his wisdom and actions how to take what is given, bring consciousness and integrity to it, discover its hidden meaning and purpose, and realize its spiritual essence.

THE HEALER AT WORK

When we bring a matured inner life to our work, we also bring calm, care, and delight. These qualities are accompanied by a sweet loving-kindness that goes out to everyone we meet. We emanate a healing presence. Every kind of work and every moment of work that is infused with consciousness can be healing to others and to ourselves. We can become a teacher of patience, care, generosity, loving-kindness, and compassion. Perhaps this *is* our actual work. Perhaps we are a healer in disguise. We can each be carriers of spirit and healers-at-work, regardless of the outer trappings of our occupation.

Your first response may be, "How can I do this?" The following is a summary of the essential steps of transformation through work.

The Preparation

We prepare for our work by first preparing our life each day. Through our daily practice, we stabilize our mind and open our heart. We then ask how our work can serve others and how we can become a healing presence for them. Throughout the day, we revisit this stillness and compassionate motivation for a few brief moments. This is particularly important when our mind becomes frenetic, our innerness has faded, our body is agitated, or our behavior is less than kind. By preparing ourselves in this way, again and again, we begin to cultivate a new relationship to our work, a relationship of soul and spirit.

The Intention

Our intention is to use work as another practice, as spirit-in-action, as engaged spirituality, as a path to integral health. Of course, the more aligned our work environment is to our goal of an integral life the easier that will be. Certainly no one should allow himself or herself to stay in a burning house, trying harder and harder to exist under impossible circumstances. But even when our job and its environment are not perfect, we can choose to take it on as a spiritual practice. That is our intention.

Transforming Our Relationship to Work

Irrespective of our work and how it comes to us, we can, much like the woodcutter, take it on as our own, bringing to it integrity, consciousness, compassion, and soul. What was previously seen as imposed is now reshaped as chosen. At first this may seem quite difficult, and we may feel much resistance. Perhaps we will only be able to do this for a few moments each day. It is important to remember our attitudes about work have been etched in stone over many years. We are taking what may seem mundane, owning it as our own, and transforming it into an act of service, artistry, and sacredness.

DISCOVERING YOUR DEEPEST CALLING

As our consciousness grows, we will progressively discover our deepest calling—a calling that best expresses our temperament, disposition, and innate talents. For some that may come early and easily while for others it may take time. I recall the advice of the poet Rainer Maria Rilke in his *Letters to a Young Poet:*

> . . . I want to beg you, as much as I can, dear sir, to be patient toward all that is unsolved in your heart and try to love the *questions themselves* like locked rooms and like books that are written in a foreign tongue. Do not seek the answers, which cannot be given you because you cannot live them. And the point is, to live every-thing. *Live* the questions now. Perhaps you will then gradually, without noticing it, live along some distant day into the answer.

And that is our direction—to live our work whatever it may be with great integrity and spirit as we move toward the consciousness and inner truth from which our authentic calling will naturally arise in its own time.

The poet Kahlil Gibran speaks to work in his masterpiece *The Prophet*. He asks us " . . . what is it to work with love?" and then he responds:

> It is to weave the cloth with threads drawn from your heart,
>   even as if your beloved were to wear that cloth.
>
> It is to build a house with affection, even as if your beloved
>   were to dwell in that house.
>
> It is to sow seeds with tenderness and reap harvest with joy,
>   as if your beloved were to eat the fruit.
>
> It is to charge all things you fashion with a breath of your spirit. . . .

Gibran asks us to work as if we were working for the beloved. But who is the beloved? In an ordinary sense we can consider the beloved to be any person for whom we have feelings of deep tenderness and affection—a friend, a family member, a spouse, or a special lover. Imagine what it would be like to work as if for the benefit and happiness of that person alone. How would it feel if work were a gracious gift we brought to our beloved each evening? What devotion and delight we would feel in our heart. Work would assume the sacredness, beauty, and connectedness of a lover meeting his or her beloved.

But there is also the other Beloved. As we journey inward to an expansive mind and an open heart, we find the inner Beloved whom we have longed for all our life—the one that is at the center of our being. This is not a personal beloved, but rather an impersonal one. It is an experience of pure awareness, an experience of the sacred. This Beloved within is the one revered and written about by the great Sufi poets Rumi, Hafez, and Kabir. It is our innate nature, our open heart, our interconnectedness with all that is, a vastness of freedom and space, a touch of the divine. To devote our work to this Beloved is to devote our work to our soul and spirit, to the divine itself.

To achieve integral life and health, work must become sacred, not when we find the right job, but right now when it is a challenge. Gibran sums up this concept in his parting advice:

> *And if you cannot work with love but only with distaste,*
> *it is better that you should leave your work*
> *and sit at the gate of the temple and take alms*
> *of those who work with joy.*

If we wish to pursue integral health and life, it is not ours to take alms at the temple gate and wonder why others find meaning and joy in their work. Integral health requires that every life challenge becomes an opportunity for practice and flourishing. All work can be a creative expression of life, a source of fulfillment, and an opportunity for service. And the same applies to each of our other outer activities. In this way, worldly life can serve as an all-encompassing practice that enriches our life, serves humankind, and simultaneously places us directly and firmly on the path toward human flourishing.

The Integral Assessment

11

We have just completed an overview of the four aspects of integral health. How do we take this theory and use it to develop a personal program? We do this by taking a careful look at our current circumstance, identifying the aspects of our life that require attention, determining the specific changes we wish to address, and establishing a program of integral practice that will promote these changes. In this way, we take an inventory of those aspects of life in which we excel and those that can use some improvement. We look for unhealthy sources of suffering and potential sources of flourishing. We use this opportunity to envision our most far-reaching possibilities and assess the obstacles to attaining them. The integral assessment is the tool we need to *choose* to transform our health and life from conventional to integral, from ordinary to precious.

THE SIX PRINCIPLES OF INTEGRAL ASSESSMENT

The following principles will help guide us:

1. *The goal of integral health is to alleviate needless suffering and promote human flourishing.* There are two criteria to use when identifying the aspects of our life that require attention:

   • Which aspects of our life are the most significant sources of distress?

   • Where is our greatest possibility for growth and development?

2. *Integral health recognizes the distinction between short-term relief of needless suffering and permanent relief.* Both must be considered when assessing our needs. For

example, heart disease may require immediate therapeutic intervention, but it may also require a long-term program of stress reduction and psychospiritual development. Irresolvable conflict in a business partnership or marriage may require an immediate upgrade of communication skills, but it also requires an understanding of the deeper sources of conflict. We must know the difference between short-term relief and long-term solutions and be able to apply each at an appropriate time.

3. *Integral health recognizes the distinction between immediate pleasure and long-term flourishing.* The first is ephemeral and acquired from outer experiences. The second is inner, self-cultivated, and sustained. Our priority is long-term flourishing. Only then can we fully enjoy worldly pleasures without the suffering of attachment and loss.

4. *Psychospiritual development is an essential component of integral health.* An expanded consciousness strengthens our capacity for attention, focuses our intention, reveals a penetrating wisdom, opens the heart, and brings to life the qualities of human flourishing. A comprehensive assessment must include this aspect of life.

5. *Integral assessment relies on deep listening and guidance.* An open, clear, and unbiased state of mind is the most effective means to an accurate and precise assessment of our health and life. This requires a mental state free of the bias of random thoughts, feelings, and images. As it is unlikely that we have fully mastered a stable calm-abiding, a wise guide may be required to assist us in listening to our inner voice and in formulating an assessment.

6. *Integral assessment addresses the aspects, levels, and lines of development that are relevant to our current circumstance.* Because dynamism is a guiding principle of integral health, our personal assessment must be modified from time to time to accommodate the changing character of our life.

LINES OF DEVELOPMENT

In Chapter 4, we introduced the four aspects of human experience—psychospiritual, biological, interpersonal, and worldly—and discussed them using a four-quadrant integral model in Chapters 6 through 10. A single line of development with four levels was shown in each of these quadrants. For example, the four levels of the biological line are anatomical body, physiological body, mind/body, and spiritual body.

I chose these representative lines of development because they are all-encompassing, relevant to health and healing, practical and possible for each of us, and serve to exemplify the evolution from body to mind to spirit that characterizes human flourishing. Now I will further enhance that model in a way that offers the opportunity for the comprehensive and detailed assessment needed to move toward integral health.

Psychospiritual Flourishing

The single line of development we used to show the progressive levels of psychospiritual development is shown in Figure 2 on page 33. In Figure 10, we replace this line with three more specific lines: conative, cognitive, and emotional.

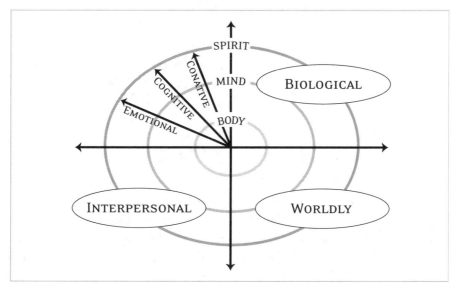

Figure 10. Psychospiritual Lines of Development

The word "conative" refers to the source and character of our motivations. We ask ourselves, "Are we motivated by survival needs, psychological needs, or spiritual imperatives?" The first source of motivation is instinctual, reactive, and ego-centered. It is usually driven by fear. The second arises from our vision and values. It is driven by culture, education, and religion. With full development, we are motivated by wisdom, wholeness, oneness, and the corresponding qualities of universal loving-kindness and compassion. What drives your life? What motivates your actions? Are you at the level of body, mind, or spirit? Is this a line of development to work on?

Now let's look at the cognitive level of development. Here the developmental sequence progresses from reactive, conditioned, and self-protective patterns to reasoning cognition that seeks a larger truth, meaning, purpose and fulfillment to the most subtle level of cognition that arrives at an understanding of the ultimate reality of self and world. What is your most stable level of cognition? Are you more reactive than you would like to be? Is your knowledge predominantly acquired through logic and reason? Or is your knowledge acquired in a non-cognitive state of pure awareness? What is the difference between information and essential truth? Which is whole and which is partial? What is important for you to address?

Finally, let's consider our emotional development. Is our emotional life dominated by uncontrolled desires, anger, fear, and other reactive emotions. Or do we live in a more neutral state where we move between afflictive emotions and transient pleasures? Finally, have we evolved to a level of stable and expansive happiness? At what level do you live? What do you need to address in this line of development?

These are the three major lines of psychospiritual development. You can assess, explore, and evolve each of these potential areas of growth and flourishing according to what is appropriate for your life and interests. Note that, in any aspect of our life, one line of development may be more evolved than another.

Biological Flourishing

Here I have selected the following three lines of development—fitness, nutrition, and self-regulation (Figure 11). The levels of nutrition progress from unconscious survival-like grasping at food to the mindful and intentional choice of a healthy diet to food choices that reflect a concern for environmental sustainability, world poverty, and animal suffering. The levels of fitness progress from exercise and movement associated with daily life to a deliberate program of fitness training that addresses specific needs such as strength, flexibility, endurance, agility, and dealing with physical disorders to a highly developed and subtle sense of body awareness. The levels of self-regulation progress from homeostasis to subtle mind/body practices to highly refined spiritual/mind/body abilities.

Other biological lines and levels of development we may wish to explore include treatment, prevention, and health promotion. How would these lines of development unfold from body to mind to spirit? Try determining the levels for each of these lines of development.

Interpersonal Flourishing

The lines of development I've selected here, shown in Figure 12, extend our previous discussion of interpersonal relationships to family and community. We can extend

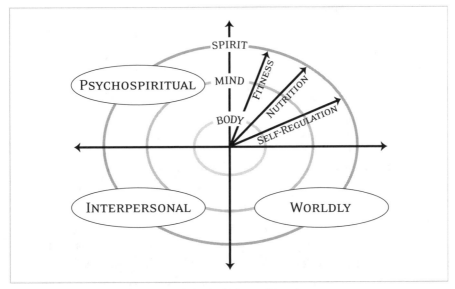

Figure 11. Biological Lines of Development

these further to coworkers, nation, and global village. Here again the movement is from body to mind to spirit as we shift from an egocentric instinctual focus on self outward toward others—from I to you to us to all of us.

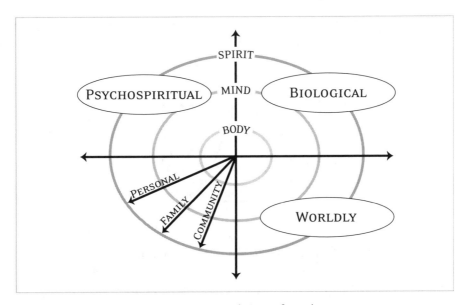

Figure 12. Interpersonal Lines of Development

Is one line of development more evolved than another? For instance, the level of development of our family life may exceed our personal life. Our community involvement may exceed our family life. Which interpersonal line of development is most urgent for you to address? Which will most benefit you in the long term? What level are you currently functioning from? What level would you like to achieve?

Worldly Flourishing

Here we focus on work, civic activism, and generativity, as shown in Figure 13. We have already explored the evolution of our work life from survival to meaning to fulfillment to service. The levels of civic and social activism evolve from a focus on day-to-day needs—for example, belonging to the parents' association at your child's school—to community and national issues to an all-inclusive global concern. Social activism can be further divided into such specific concerns as environmental issues, health policy, educational initiatives, social justice, and so on. Here again each area will have its levels of development. For example, environmental activism can reach from home recycling to spearheading a campaign against global warming. If this line of development is appropriate for you, there is much to choose from.

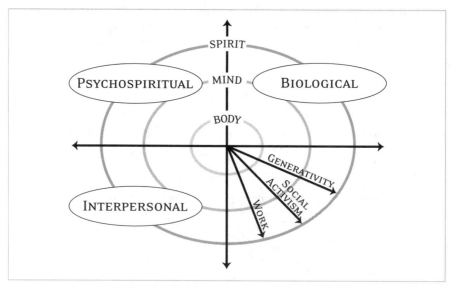

Figure 13. Worldly Lines of Development

Our third line of development, generativity, is the effort we make to teach others what we have learned. This intergenerational transmission of knowledge, skills, values, and wisdom will serve future generations. It may occur through individual mentoring, organizational development, or promotion of social policy. Generativity can occur at any age but expands and matures over a lifetime. For example, the high school senior can help the freshman, the more experienced worker can assist the novice, or the elder can mentor younger colleagues.

OUR PERSONAL ASSESSMENT

In Figure 14, we see the full spectrum of aspects, lines, and levels in all four quadrants. It should be clear by now that our development is uneven. We have different talents, capacities, abilities, training, and upbringing. As a result, one or more lines of development may have received a better start or more attention than another. We may excel in fitness, be average in nutrition, relatively unconscious in our words and actions, great with our family but unable to attain personal intimacy, a star at work but uninvolved with the larger world. The path to integral health requires that we at least become aware of the sources of needless suffering, distress, and dissatisfaction and the possible sources of future development and flourishing.

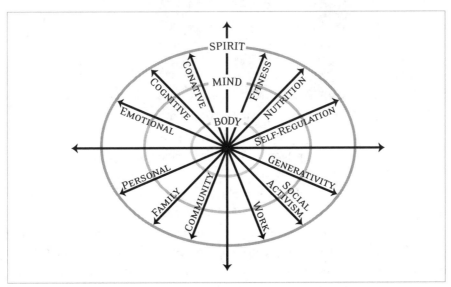

Figure 14. Aspects, Lines, and Levels of Development

Integral health does not require that we develop fully in every way. This is not our goal. We have different needs throughout our life cycle, varying life circumstances, and even different destinies. Any one line of development taken to its final goal, realized in its fully evolved movement from body to mind to spirit, can lead to human flourishing. That works because all lines and levels of development are inextricably interconnected. Health, happiness, and wholeness are arrived at through our own unique path. The only constant is the need for psychospiritual development.

Ken Wilber, who developed integral theory, suggests another way of quantifying our integral status, as shown in Figure 15. Here we can use a bar graph to plot our movement along lines of development so we see the changes we make over time. We can assess our current level of integral development, set goals for the future, or add further lines and levels in accord with our needs and goals.

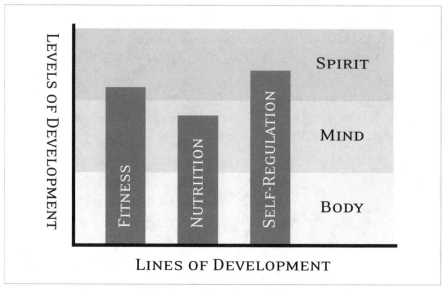

Figure 15. A Sample Biograph

We can further personalize this graphic by noting specific milestones in our integral development. Consider the nutrition line and ask yourself the following questions: To what extent do my eating patterns continue to be driven by habit? When did I develop mindfulness about nutrition? How has this awareness unfolded over time? Is my concern about physiological balance, immune-system enhancement, vitality, inner calmness, or global food chains? Where am I coming from and where am I going? What are my priorities? What practices (we will explore integral practice in the next chapter) will assist with this shift? Create a line of development in your journal. Establish goals and timetables and identify practices that can take you toward your goal.

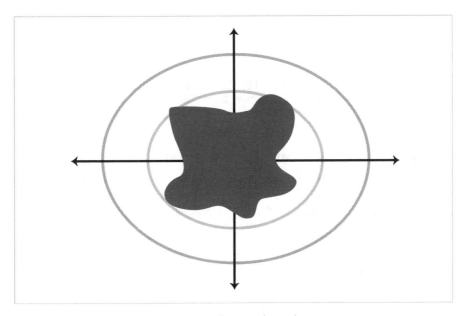

Figure 16. Overall Integral Development

Another way of looking at our overall circumstances is shown in Figure 16. Here we can see the larger picture and compare development in the different aspects of our life and across the various lines and levels of development. This dynamic graph will change over time. There is no one perfect contour. There is only the increasing awareness of where you are in the integral process and where you would like to go. Don't be surprised if you find yourself overdeveloped in one area and underdeveloped in another. That is the usual case. The point here is to become integral and balanced.

Here's an example of the assessment process. Several years ago a woman came to me about a severe case of ulcerative colitis. She had been receiving medical treatment for several years and was now in remission. She requested my assistance in preventing further recurrences. We began with several minutes of silence. I then listened openly and empathically to the history of her illness, exploring its sources in each of the four aspects of her life. There was much to relate: the medical treatments, the interpersonal stress that was a trigger, her psychospiritual development, which was a major factor in her troubled relationships, and issues with work and career. There was no single cause for her illness.

The discussion took about two hours. At the end, a sense of silence enveloped the room. We closed our eyes again, and I guided her in contemplation until she arrived at an inner stillness and peace. I then asked, "Do you think the colitis could recur in the presence of such an inner state?" She considered this for several moments and said, "No, definitely no." As we continued the meditation, I pointed out to her that this was her inner essence: peace, clarity, spaciousness, and ease, which were always within her. She began to cry tears of relief. I offered to teach her how to access this inner space through contemplative practice. In this way, we completed an initial assessment and an introduction to contemplative practice.

We opened our eyes and continued to review the areas of concern, assessing the aspects of her life that required attention and the specific issues that needed to be addressed. We settled on a preliminary plan that would aid in both preventing recurrence and promoting well-being. We agreed she would continue her medical care, explore the difficulties in her relationships and the related psychological concerns, address her diet and supplement it with certain nutrients, and begin contemplative practice. I suggested readings, instructed her on contemplative practice, and discussed several mind/ body exercises. We agreed to speak again the following week. On her way out the door, after we had spent three hours together, she expressed a sense of hope and relief.

This was the beginning of a year of exploration and growth in which she discovered new understandings, developed essential skills through practice, and identified important resources. The original focus on colitis subtly shifted to a focus on integral development—attaining greater health, happiness, and wholeness. This, she felt, was not only the best preventive regimen, but it also brought meaning and purpose to her life. Slowly my role diminished as she became increasingly capable of assessing her life and moving it forward.

NOTES FROM A FELLOW TRAVELER

Without knowing which aspects of our life to work with we cannot effectively choose the right practices or efficiently progress toward integral health and healing. Where we place our effort depends on what is relevant to our life, what aligns with our abilities, and what is actually possible given our circumstances. But it's important to remember, as in the example above, that disease and health have their roots in each of the four aspects of our life. So we must be holistic in our assessment even though at any one time we may choose to act in only one area of life.

Using my understanding of the four quadrants, lines, and levels of development, I find it helpful to begin a formal assessment of myself while in a contemplative state. First, I cultivate a still and silent mind. Next, I focus my full attention on the four quadrants of the integral map. (You can make an image of the map or simply have a sense of it.) I then take inventory of the four aspects of my life and determine which area needs attention.

Depending on what's going on in my life at that time, I might choose to focus on any of the four quadrants and then fine-tune this by identifying the specific lines of development I would like to address. This could be personal relationships, emotional development, fitness, work, or another concern. I then visualize the leap to the next level of development. What practices will this require? What problems will I resolve? What new abilities will I develop? How will this contribute to integral health?

Another approach is to identify any urgent area of distress. It's important to address that concern in all the related quadrants, lines, and levels. At which level of development am I stuck or out of balance? When I find it, I can then address it through practice. For example, if I were diagnosed with an illness, I would consider how each aspect of my life impacts on that problem. Do I seek medical treatment to deal with the mechanics of the disease, expand my consciousness to help address its deeper sources, seek the support of close relationships, or develop self-regulation skills? Which are most appropriate and in which order? I jot down a few notes and recheck my observations a few more times. I want to be both accurate and precise before undertaking integral practice.

Close your eyes and let's try this together. Rest into the ease and stillness of your mind and body, releasing all mental activity. When quiet, ask yourself, "What aspect of my life—psychospiritual, biological, interpersonal, or worldly—is the source of difficulty and suffering?" Focus on this one area. What line of development is most essential for me at this time? What is my current level of development and what can I aim for? This is the first aspect of assessment. You may explore this over several days or weeks.

Return to recenter in stillness. We'll now shift from a focus on healing to a focus on promoting integral development. You may now ask, "What area of my life is ready for growth and development? Is it the same area that also needs healing or is it another area? What would the next level of development look like? This is the second aspect of assessment. You may wish to jot down a few thoughts in your journal.

If I am with a wise guide, I use one of these approaches while in silent communion. I slowly share my assessment and then listen as the clean and polished mirror of my guide as he or she reflects back what he or she has heard. Have I been clear and unbiased in my assessment? Am I taking on too much or too little? Together we share a community of truth and support whose aim is integral health and healing.

As we become progressively more experienced with the integral process, our enhanced awareness itself will serve as an informal and ongoing assessment tool. Each day if I wish, I can ask myself: "How have I handled this or that experience? At what level was I functioning? In what way could I improve my attitude or actions? How can I be a better person contributing to a better world? How can I move my life toward a more sustained health, happiness, and wholeness?" With time I will no longer think in fragmented ways, speak or act as if I am disconnected from the whole, limit myself to an underdeveloped consciousness, or view my life from the narrow perspective of ordinary health. I will think, feel, speak, and act from an integral perspective.

It's important to remember that it's always possible to have a peak/peek experience in any one line of development. That could be a moment of unity consciousness attained through nature, meditation, or sexuality; an extraordinary sense of wellness and peace experienced at the apex of adventure or fitness; or an all-encompassing universal loving-kindness that spontaneously arises from deep love. But these are temporary states. We are not in control of this glimpse. The circumstance is. So if we want more, we have to go back to the situation, and slowly we become attached and addicted to it. We don't gain freedom and human flourishing. We become slaves to the outer sources of these peak/peek experiences.

The full flowering of these levels of achievement—sustained health, happiness, and wholeness—will not occur until we prepare the ground and carefully ripen our lives. When we do that, the results will be permanent and irreversible like an etching in stone.

An accurate and honest assessment of our actual level of development will allow us to plan for the future. We will be able to choose and apply the most appropriate integral practice toward our goal of ending needless suffering, enhancing recovery from disease, and promoting authentic well-being. In this way, integral assessment helps us get from one level of development to another, progressively moving us toward our precious goal of human flourishing.

Integral Practice

12

Without integral practice, we experience only a portion of the health that is available to us. It is the portion that is in accord with the beliefs, values, and practices of our culture. However, if we gather together the wisdom and methods developed throughout time and across diverse cultures, we will gain an understanding of the human possibility that far exceeds the vision, knowledge, and approaches of any one culture.

In this way, we will uncover a vision of health, happiness, and wholeness that is comprehensive in that it covers all aspects of human experience, sustained in that it is immune to outer adversities, and expansive in its reach for extended capacities and human flourishing. Never before have humans been able to access, catalogue, and utilize the scope of knowledge that is now available to assist us in attaining a far-reaching health. Our access to the accomplishments of diverse cultures; new and advanced research into somatic, sensory, cognitive, and contemplative capacities; and an interest in integral theory enable us to envision health that reflects the full flourishing of the human possibility.

What we are discovering is that all our "normal" capacities, when addressed with intention and proper training, can be enhanced and extended—including our capacity for health. Our ability for self-reflection can become a highly refined contemplative consciousness. Our capacity for romantic love can be matured and developed into a profound universal loving-kindness. The ability to move our muscles and walk down the street can be evolved into the finely tuned dexterity of a master pianist. Our innate mind/body interconnectedness can develop into a highly refined ability for self-regulation. Our five senses can function with a sensitivity and capacity that is called extrasensory perception. Muscular strength and flexibility can be enhanced through intense training. The entrepreneurial mind that has created great centers of wealth is also capable of evolving the inner wisdom and compassion that can bring an end to poverty and war. By expanding our normal human capacities into extraordinary ones, we can arrive at radiant health of body, mind, and spirit.

THE EIGHT PRINCIPLES OF INTEGRAL PRACTICE

How do we find radiant health? We do that by choosing the broader integral vision, assessing our life from an integral perspective, and incorporating integral practices into our daily routine. Integral practice is the path to this expansive vision, and it is composed of a series of activities of body, mind, and spirit that grow our capacity in each of the four aspects of life. The abundance of practices that contribute to integral health and healing are not found in any one culture or in any one discipline. We must gather them together from diverse cultures and multiple disciplines.

Some practices are all-encompassing. For example, contemplative practices simultaneously catalyze our capacities in all or multiple areas of our life. These cross-training practices offer us a full integral workout. Other practices tend to affect only one or perhaps two aspects of our life. These targeted practices are not integral in nature. But when they are integrated with other practices, they become part of a comprehensive integral process.

Because we are defining a new approach to health and healing, it is important to establish a set of principles that can help us understand and distinguish the essential characteristics of integral practice. The tendency of our culture is for those who want to profit from quick fixes or easy answers to co-opt and then dilute new approaches. As a result, efforts to establish a new approach are often contaminated early on by well-intentioned but mistaken advocates, commercial interests, and opportunistic pretenders. So the potential impact of a new approach is easily and subtly undermined. In order to defend and maintain its integrity, we must define the eight essential characteristics of integral practice.

1. *All integral practices must have as their final aim the evolution of our knowledge, capacity, and abilities beyond what is now considered normal.* For this to occur, our practices must address and support each aspect of life with the goal of fully realizing all levels of human potential available to the individual given his or her life circumstances, such as age, temperament, stage of life, existing commitments, native capacities, and general level of health. The evolution of this potential is from body

to mind to spirit. Previous, limited understandings of health, disease, aging, and death must be abandoned.

2. *All integral practices must be supported by inner development.* Contemplative practice is an essential component of all approaches to integral health. Only through an expanded consciousness can we transcend the emotional wounds from childhood, reactive patterns, conditioned beliefs, and limited understandings that will otherwise undermine our efforts. Mental training and subtle consciousness provide the space, clarity, wisdom, and attention that is a fundamental requirement for the success of other practices. Only through an expanded consciousness can we complete the movement from body to mind to spirit in each aspect of our life.

3. *All integral practices must be infused with an aspiration for loving-kindness.* Universal loving-kindness is an embrace of life that softens the mind and opens the heart. It subdues our uncontrolled impulses and passions, diminishes the grip of our ego, and conveys a larger meaning to our life. It further assists us in gaining the good will, encouragement, and support of others. When our practices are suffused with loving-kindness, their very character changes and their transformative powers are enhanced.

4. *All integral practices must be infused with virtue.* Courage, creativity, patience, discipline, perseverance, openness, confidence, and enthusiasm are some of the character traits that fuel our practice. Without these human qualities, our practices become mere methods that seek only limited, immediate results. The achievement of integral health develops over a long period of time marked by spurts of activity and periods of rest, by moments of enthusiasm and moments of discouragement. Unless we have the strength of character that can maintain our vision and sustain our efforts, we will not be able to stay the course.

5. *All integral practices must be tailored to the individual's needs.* We are each born with a unique disposition, temperament, and life circumstance. As a result, we have our distinct way of moving toward integral health and choosing and using the practices that best suit our particular style. Unlike the methods used for conventional health, no one approach fits all. Our capacity, and abilities change with age and circumstance. Throughout our life cycle, each of us must be able to adapt specific practices to our own needs and be flexible in reshaping them when necessary. Practitioners must be even more flexible when responding to their clients' needs. They cannot automatically reach into their tool kit and choose from the available remedies, therapies, and approaches. Any one practitioner's tool kit is too limited for an

integral approach. Integral practices must be based on an individual's specific needs and the totality of available resources.

6. *Integral practice requires more than one helper or mentor.* Because the integral approach is broad-based and relies on practices that touch each aspect of our experience, no one practitioner has access to or even knowledge of the full range of practices. What will be necessary in the future is more broadly based, multidisciplined healers and healing centers that follow an integral vision and incorporate a well-integrated array of practices. This may include individuals uniquely trained as integral resource counselors who are knowledgeable about a wide variety of integral approaches, familiar with related books, seminars, and online information, and capable of tailoring person-centered programs. However, we must be careful when choosing our teachers, practices, and retreat facilities. The integrity of the integral vision and of these principles must be carefully preserved. Unfortunately, some practitioners and centers may not necessarily live up to their label.

7. *Integral practice requires that we take responsibility for our own development.* Because no one practitioner can encompass all the knowledge and capacities we need, and even less can he or she be fully attuned to our personal situation, we must become "general contractors." Assuming overall responsibility for integral health will help us build autonomy, skillfulness, discernment, discipline, and the capacity for improvisation. As managers of our own integral process, we will be able to undertake an integral assessment and know when to move in one direction or another, when to stay put in a practice, when to reshape it, and when to let go. We have the best chance of getting it right and most efficiently and effectively advancing on our integral path.

8. *Integral practice emphasizes activities that are broad-based, simultaneously touching multiple aspects of our life.* For example, contemplative practices that range from formal meditation to active meditations such as tai chi still our mind and expand our consciousness. They harmonize our body/mind/spirit, enhance the quality of our relationships, and support a more effective presence in worldly life.

Never before have we had as much access to as many practices as we do now. We can pick and choose from an abundance of well-developed disciplines. Master practitioners speak at conferences, publish books, and record videos, audiotapes, and DVDs. We can enter into online dialogues with experts through the ease of worldwide communication. We are just beginning to explore how to mix and match the abundance of cross-cultural resources. This will allow each of us to find the correct practices to meet our individual needs. Though we may have less guidance than we might like, we are really pioneers with far more opportunity and access to resources than has previously been possible in any one culture.

But this wealth of opportunity also brings with it a set of obstacles that we must be aware of, overcome, and, if possible, avoid. Too much information can confuse and stall our efforts. Discernment and focus are essential. We must learn who and what we can rely on. Superficial approaches and claims must be seen for what they are. The gulf between disciplines and specialists may impede integral understandings and advice. Here again we must do the best we can to organize and personalize our integral approach. Self-proclaimed "gurus" who seek to narrow our vision to their singular approach may be quite convincing, but if we follow their principles, we will soon discover they are not integral in their understanding.

Finally, we must accept that irrespective of the cultural shifts going on all around us, adopting integral practices means we will be working against our culture. There is no health insurance to cover the cost of integral practices and often little support from family and close friends. We may have to look toward like-minded individuals and communities and schedule regular integral retreats for encouragement and support. But in the end we must accept our role as pioneers and the adventure that entails with all its glory and uncertainties. We are moving into the future rather than hanging out in the past.

DESIGNING YOUR INTEGRAL PRACTICE

There are two ways to approach integral practice. The first is to combine a series of practices into a single program, which we will call an Integral Practice Program. It is important to recognize that such a carefully organized program is more efficient and effective that any one practice in the program and more far-reaching than the sum of its individual components. The second approach is to transform our routine daily activities and interactions into integral practices. This approach is called life-as-practice. Taking this approach requires considerable skill. We are not always involved in programmed activities, but we are always involved in daily life. So if we transform the activities of daily life into integral practices, we will be practicing all the time. In this way, we can gradually incorporate the integral vision into our daily life and slowly blur the boundary between our formal program and life itself.

The first approach will shift and change as we continue along the path. The second will remain the same in principle while encompassing more and more of our daily activities over time. Combining the two will result in a more efficient, effective, and integrated program.

Each of the approaches shares a key element. Because contemplative practices are the most effective, efficient, cross-training integral practices, they must be a central component of both approaches. Contemplative practice anchors, steadies, and orients the entire integral process. It provides a backdrop of ongoing psychospiritual development that assures the integral process is holistic in addressing each aspect of life *and* evolutionary in its final aim of human flourishing.

The Integral Practice Program

An Integral Practice Program is a fully integrated and coordinated series of practices. We create an integral program by combining a series of practices that broaden the reach of any one practice and then anchor and fuel them with contemplative practice. There are many varieties of contemplative practice. They may include Christian centering prayer, mindfulness meditation, focused attention, devotional chanting, and visualization. We can choose whichever meets our beliefs, needs, and style.

Figure 17 provides a preliminary diagram of the types of activities we can consider when putting together an integral program. To remind us of each aspect of our life as we develop our program, these are arranged by quadrants as shown in previous

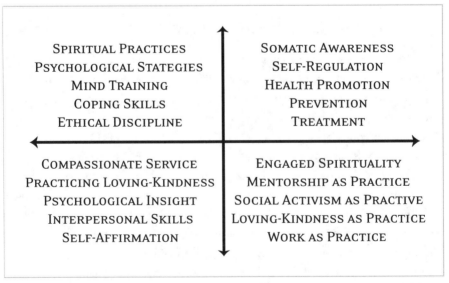

SPIRITUAL PRACTICES
PSYCHOLOGICAL STATEGIES
MIND TRAINING
COPING SKILLS
ETHICAL DISCIPLINE

SOMATIC AWARENESS
SELF-REGULATION
HEALTH PROMOTION
PREVENTION
TREATMENT

COMPASSIONATE SERVICE
PRACTICING LOVING-KINDNESS
PSYCHOLOGICAL INSIGHT
INTERPERSONAL SKILLS
SELF-AFFIRMATION

ENGAGED SPIRITUALITY
MENTORSHIP AS PRACTICE
SOCIAL ACTIVISM AS PRACTIVE
LOVING-KINDNESS AS PRACTICE
WORK AS PRACTICE

Figure 17. Developing an Integral Practice Program

figures. Within each quadrant there are a series of broad categories that can be further expanded into a variety of targeted practices. For example, prevention strategies in the upper right-hand quadrant may include activities related to fitness, nutrition, risk-reduction, stress management, laboratory screening, and genetic monitoring. Social activism in the lower right-hand quadrant may include integral approaches to environmental concerns, social policy, or worksite wellness.

We are each responsible for setting up our own integral program and finding the proper helpers. We must first examine our life through our integral assessment and determine which aspects require the most attention. This is a critical task. It requires deep listening that goes far beyond our surface needs. We have already discussed how we can use contemplative practice to develop this skill. And we have recommended finding a skillful helper who can listen with us from a still space for however long we need help.

We then need to do research to determine which programs will be best suited to our temperament and level of development. Because the resources available to us may be confusing, contradictory, anecdotal, and at times commercially motivated, we will need time, patience, and discernment. I cannot stress enough the importance of giving this process the attention it deserves. In consultation with others, we can carefully select an integral practice that will provide us with the skills and capacities that address our needs. We then combine these practices into an integrated program, one practice at a time, carefully checking to see that each practice still seems right after we try it. We want to choose the proper practices so we can move forward as efficiently and effectively as possible. Discrimination, an open mind, and the willingness to shift directions as needed are essential. Finally, we must remember to anchor our integral program with daily contemplative practice.

When choosing a practice, it is as important to choose the practitioner as it is to choose the practice. In actuality, it may be even more important. Why is that? Very talented integral practitioners will use their practice as an entrance into a larger engagement with life. Irrespective of their specific training, they will listen carefully to you and your needs and place this above loyalty to any one method. Their priority must be to assist you to develop an integrated, far-reaching approach to your health and life. Through their presence, skill, deep listening, and loving-kindness such healers act as midwife to your hidden potential. If you find such a wise healer, you are investing more in the healer and less so in his or her approach. Practitioners and practices are plentiful; wise healers are rare. The investment in a wise healer is the most important investment you can make.

Finally, we must learn to carefully and skillfully monitor our program and our progress. Remember that one of the principles of integral healing is dynamism. We change and our needs change. A practice that may be very helpful for a period of time may lose its value over time. When we grow and have maximized the value of a practice, we need to find a new practice that will take us to the next level. Likewise, another area of our life may become a new area for growth. Perhaps we start a new relationship. Working on our life through a relationship may now be the way to go. The same can be said of a new position at work. So another round of assessment, research, and consultation may be at hand. With each new step we take, we are learning how to become our own healer in a new creative adventure. Rest assured, this process takes time and patience.

In the previous chapter, I gave the example of a woman who came to me with a history of recurrent ulcerative colitis. After the initial assessment process, we settled on a preliminary program of practice that included contemplative practice, nutrition, and mind/body exercises. These were practices that she did on her own. But we also addressed her personal relationships, which were a source of mental distress and obvious triggers of colitis. We identified a program of reading, reviewed the loving-kindness practice, and agreed on specific ways she could work with her relationships each day. This latter aspect of her program uses her life-as-practice. Using life-as-practice is the second aspect of an integral practice program.

Life-as-Practice

When we seek to use our life as practice, we discover there are as many possible practices as there are people. A poet enters contemplation through poetry. Creativity can become his or her practice. The same can be said of a sculptor, painter, musician, composer, writer, or any other artist. A plumber, electrician, gardener, doctor, or lawyer can, much like the woodcarver, similarly transform his or her craft into an integral practice. We have already considered two examples of this—the transformation of our relationships and our work into integral practices.

In this way, every act, experience, word, and person can become a practice. But the transformation from routine activity to integral practice does not occur automatically. It must be cultivated. We have to infuse our daily activity with the awareness, consciousness, and loving-kindness that arise from contemplative practice. We have to shift out of automatic to find the essence and healing potential that is hidden in what seems routine. We have to pay attention and act out of awareness and intention. That is why we emphasize that the effort to use activities of daily life as a practice requires that we first ground ourselves in contemplative practice. For example, we discussed how to apply this transformative process to work in Chapter 10. It might be helpful to review this step-by-step process.

I have included a brief survey of some common activities and transitions of life to show how they can be transformed into integral practices. They are just examples. All aspects of our life—whatever we are doing, whomever we are meeting—can be brought into the integral path. That is our aim. An integral life is not ultimately found in formal practice. It is found in living integrally day by day.

- *Nature.* Nature mirrors the wholeness, harmony, and peace that reside within each of us. It helps us remember our essence. It has a special way of stilling the mind, allowing us a glimpse of the ever-present simplicity and beauty of life. That's why our communion with nature should not go unnoticed or become little more than a pleasurable distraction from urban life. To turn this communion into an integral experience, we must deepen it through contemplative practice.

  The next time you commune with nature take it as an opportunity to experience and explore your still mind. Notice its pristine awareness and simple presence. What is happening to your usual mental movements? Are you grasping at them or allowing them to come and go? Do you notice the vastness, timelessness, and spaciousness of the subtle aspect of the mind? Can you see the difference between the still and moving mind? Is there anything outside of yourself that can offer the peace, happiness, and wholeness of the subtle mind? To bring awareness to your experience in nature is to transform your communion with nature into an integral practice. Nature becomes your teacher rather than your addiction.

- *The creative arts.* Art was a daily experience at the Aesclepian temples. May it be the same for us. What is possible when art becomes an integral experience rather than an entertaining pleasure? Edvard Munch's masterpiece *The Scream* can connect us to our deepest and most afflictive emotions. René Magritte's paintings shock our mind into the unfamiliar, interrupting our usual mental activity and thrusting us into the experience of the unknown. Mark Rothko takes us directly to the contemplative mind. Alex Grey offers a visual view of transcendence. Dance inspires us with its harmony, beauty, balance, and disciplined ease. Drama, be it Sophocles' Oedipus trilogy or Arthur Miller's *Death of a Salesman,* teaches us about humanity's existential condition. Music, whether an English madrigal, a Mozart opera, African drums, a Peruvian wind pipe, or devotional chanting, transports our mind/body into unexplored inner realms. Reading poetry, fiction, and essays introduces us to new ideas and helps us examine old feelings and experience new ones. Each of these creative art forms can challenge us to explore, examine, and further develop our life.

There is yet another way in which the creative experience can serve as an integral practice. When we are fully absorbed into music, dance, or art, this focused concentration brings the active mind to stillness. Similar to our experience in nature, we are lifted out of our usual mental state. If we become aware of the clarity and stillness of our mind, our focus will shift from the art to our subtle mind. There we can experience and explore its unique qualities.

Whether art catalyzes a deeper examination of our life, allows a further experience of our subtle mind, or both, we are embodying the artist's intent. The artist wishes to take you deeper into life, below the surface to its essence. If we are willing to travel with the artist, we can experience the depths of both art and life. Art can become an integral practice, and an integral practice carefully cultivated can itself become an art.

- *Sexuality.* With great awareness and proper intent, sexuality can also be transformed into an integral practice. It can enhance intimacy and take you toward a spiritual union. If you can stay clear and present during the rising bliss of sexual experience, you will discover that at the moment preceding and extending through orgasm time stops, the mind stops, control stops, the I disappears, and you are involuntarily propelled into an experience of oneness and sheer presence. You are no longer enclosed in your small self. Only oneness is possible. If you can hold pure awareness rather than becoming lost in lust, ordinary life and sexuality are transcended, and you are privileged to taste the simplicity and profundity of spirit itself.

  It is no surprise that the singular symbol the East has chosen to represent the state of divine union is the image of sexual union. This is not about sexuality as we know and indulge in it, but rather it is about the sacred and divine. It is not an early practice. It is a demanding practice that follows the development of a stable and inward knowing mind. Those who have accomplished it have raised sexuality to the level of high practice.

- *Other people.* Personal interactions provide the most ever-present and important opportunities for practice. They can be both teacher and teaching. Interacting with others, whether at home, at work, or in community activities, gives us the opportunity to explore our disturbing emotions and practice loving-kindness, generosity, patience, and compassion. To transform our routine personal interactions into practice requires mindfulness, intention, and a desire to learn from another.

  With each person we meet, we need to take time, listen carefully, create a heart connection, and act with skill. For example, if we are in a circumstance in which we feel anger, we can stop, practice patience, see the suffering of this person, look into the beauty of their innate soul, witness our projections and reactivity, and bring forth care and compassion as a needed antidote to our anger. If we become jealous of another, we can ask ourselves why we cannot rejoice in their accomplishments. Our daily interactions provide endless opportunities for profound integral practice. We can combine many practices into one.

• *Disease and aging.* Disease and aging can lead to resignation, resentment, and despair, or they can be transformed into integral practice. Most of us ask, "How can such a difficult experience become an opening?" The experience of disease and the recognition of aging suddenly bring daily life and its routines to a halt. Where there was no time to spare, there is now time. Surface concerns give way to more profound ones. Past and future collapse into the present moment. The mind itself can become more focused and aware of life.

   The great scholar and philosopher Joseph Campbell said it well when he said we spend our life climbing up a ladder, and finally, when we reach the top and look over the wall, we discover that we have placed our ladder against the wrong wall. Disease and aging offer us a quick trip up this ladder. They confront us with questions about meaning, purpose, and value. When deeply felt, these challenges allow us to see what is true and important in life. There is an immediacy to these issues that drives inner exploration. They give us a chance to move our ladder to the right wall that leads to an authentic life. With the help of the proper teachers, we can discover the vast possibilities of integral health in the midst of the growing limitations of our physical body. Disease and aging provide powerful integral practices.

• *Death.* We come to the final opportunity to evolve our life when we confront death itself. Impending death can take us very rapidly toward the revelation of the inner world and its profound mysteries. When we are freed from the restraints of the physical body, its senses and cognition, we can see beyond. The wise ones tell us that if we can bring focused awareness to the death process, we can directly experience the most subtle aspects of the mind. They say death can give rise to a very subtle and luminous consciousness that alone knows and survives this final life transition. A profound healing occurs.

BOTTOM-UP, TOP-DOWN HEALTH AND HEALING

As we can see from these examples, every aspect of life can be transformed into an integral practice. When we combine a coordinated series of formal practices with our strategy to use life as a practice, we have a powerful twofold approach that leads us directly along the path to integral health and well-being. Our mind will still, our heart will open, wisdom will flourish, and we will discover the truth and treasures of life.

But that's not all. There are actually two ways of achieving human flourishing—from the bottom-up and from the top-down. Throughout this book and in this chapter, we have discussed the bottom-up developmental approach. The top-down experience of transformation is quite different. Here we are referring to a transformative change that is full and complete at the moment it happens without any clear preceding cause. It is as if a force not previously known to us reveals a profoundly larger knowledge. This often occurs around major transitions of life such as during times of unrelenting suffering, healing, painful loss, life-threatening disease, and death. It is rare, but when it occurs, it is permanent and dramatic. It is life changing. We call this quick top-down path *grace*. For most of our life we work from the bottom up and give thanks if the mystery of grace enters our life.

It is my hope that integral practice will become the mainstay of your quest for a more expansive and comprehensive health. The integral vision is large enough to embrace all approaches to health, and yet it is innovative enough to transcend their limitations. But this matter is not yet settled. There is much room for us to grow and mature this approach, and each one of us can contribute to this unfolding if we choose to undertake this lifelong adventure.

The Four
Essential Points

Throughout this book we've seen extensive evidence that a new level of health and well-being is about to emerge in human life. Its character cannot be fully known through traditional inquiries of medical science or those of any other discipline. What is required is an integral inquiry that explores, catalogs, and integrates the vast cross-cultural reservoir of knowledge that bears on human health. This knowledge spans the full spectrum of the human experience, including medical science, contemplative practices, traditional healing methods, psychological theory, anthropological studies, high-end athletic performance, self-regulation, cognitive training, psychic research, and mystical unitary experiences. This all-encompassing integral perspective is the foundation for an epochal shift that will result in an entirely new vision of health that we call human flourishing.

As individuals we will play a role by elevating our sights toward this transcendent shift. We do this by choosing and embodying an integral vision that is holistic, evolutionary, and far reaching. In so doing, we cultivate an aspiration that is equal to our possibilities. We aspire toward a healthier and happier personal life and extend this aspiration toward all humankind. Intention, practice, and perseverance will allow us to realize integral health in this lifetime, and we can use our remaining years to serve our troubled world. In this way, we become an expression of the future and a model and mentor for others.

We must stress again that integral health does not begin on the mountaintops. We pursue it in the valley, in the midst of our daily life. We look up to the pinnacle of achievement to be inspired and assured. And, in an act of deserved reverence, we thank those special ones who have taken the full journey and shown us what is possible. But these rare individuals have devoted their entire lives to this one lofty goal. Their path, as ours, also began with intention, practice, and perseverance—the simple daily work of an integral approach. All they ask is that we discard our conditioned and culturally based ideas, turn ourselves toward what is now possible for humanity, and begin to take the small but essential steps outlined in this book. If you do so, you will discover that the valley, the foothills, the ascent, and the summit are all magnificent.

The masters constantly warn us about the strength of our inner conditioning and our innate tendency to fall back onto the known, well-traveled, comfortable path. One of their most powerful antidotes to this tendency is to teach and reteach the same essential points. With each teaching, those with more cultivated and motivated minds are further primed to hear their message at subtler levels. So each retelling is in fact a new opportunity to find deeper meanings, to affirm our choice, and to inspire our actions. The following four essential points distilled from the preceding chapters define, distinguish, and illuminate the path to integral health and life. They highlight and add subtlety to what we have learned and explored. Studying them focuses our attention on the main issues, clears up any lingering doubts or confusion, and sets us forthrightly on the path to integral health.

THE FIRST POINT: THE TRUTH OF HEALTH

There are two aspects of health—ordinary, or relative, health and integral, or ultimate, health.

Ordinary, or relative, health is based upon our biology. It is our conventional understanding of health. We are healthy when our body is free of the signs and symptoms of disease or disability, and unhealthy when they are present. This is what is meant by relative health—it is relative to our biological functioning. Health based on the condition of the body is always in flux, uncertain, temporary, and invariably deteriorates with aging and imminent death. In fact, ordinary health changes moment to moment as our body subtly undergoes the less apparent and subtler aspects of aging.

The second aspect of health is integral, or ultimate, health. It is based on our level of consciousness. We are healthy when our mind is both free of mental afflictions and suffering and when we experience an enduring well-being, happiness, and wholeness that is independent of our biology and outer circumstances. Integral, or ultimate, health is sustained regardless of the adversities of life, aging, and death. It is intentional, self-cultivated, and flourishes over time. This aspect of health is the unique and precious possibility of human life.

Both of these aspects of health are essential. Without biological well-being, it would be far more difficult to evolve our consciousness, which is the basis of an integral, or ultimate, health. In fact, this is why our body is so precious. It is not because of the momentary and deceptive pleasures that it appears to provide, but rather because of the opportunity our biology offers for the development of a far-reaching, profound, and sustained integral and ultimate health of body, mind, and spirit.

So we must honor both aspects of health but know their differences. We must support our biological health so that it can serve as a platform for the development of our mind and the evolution of our consciousness. The development of our consciousness then becomes the basis for the highest and most meaningful form of human health. This integral health of human flourishing embraces a conventional physical health while transcending its temporal, circumstantial, and biological limitations.

THE SECOND POINT: THE TRUTH OF HUMAN FLOURISHING

Human flourishing is a profound, sustained, and self-cultivated health, happiness, and wholeness. It is an innate and natural human potential that each and every one of us can actualize. It is the noble aim and final fulfillment of human life. Its attainment is the highest meaning of human life

The qualities of human flourishing can be fully and permanently experienced only if we prepare the proper foundation and steadily progress in our development from body to mind to spirit. But like the flower encoded in the seed, gold obscured by encrusted stone, the sun concealed by dense clouds, or the butter latent in milk, they are obstructed but nevertheless they are always and already in us. Although we do not yet have full access to these qualities, we can get a glimpse of them, and this taste can inspire and motivate us. There are four ways we can get this taste.

1. As noted earlier in this book, we are able to catch brief glimpses of these qualities when there's a momentary break in ordinary consciousness. This break offers a peak/peek experience of life's essence that lies unseen beneath our day-to-day routines. We experience a cessation of mental movements, an openness, peace, timelessness, and selflessness. However, these tantalizing glimpses are quite ephemeral and cannot be sustained without further development. They fall short of the sustained wisdom, loving-kindness, compassion, and delight that emerge with full development.

2. We can experience and feel the quality of this level of life by being face-to-face with those who have arrived at this final aim. We look into their eyes, feel their presence, experience their loving-kindness, admire their wisdom, and envy their imperturbable inner peace. We feel inspired and assured that this is indeed a possibility for each of us as it has been for them. If we have the fortunate opportunity, we may request that they assist us as a guide and teacher.

3. We can also intuit these possibilities by becoming aware of the yearning of our spirit and soul. We all know this inner longing. It keeps us searching, though it too often manifests in mistaken ways. It is driven by the faint but certain remembrance of our authentic, natural home, which is human flourishing. This remembrance is our glimpse.

4. Finally, we can experience the qualities of human flourishing if we enter the integral path and undertake the practices that will expand consciousness. This process will gradually provide us with the insight and development needed to penetrate life's surface and see directly into the essence of our own nature. Then we can experience and know intimately, directly, and permanently the human qualities of sustained health, happiness, and wholeness.

If we want to achieve this higher goal, we will have to overcome obstacles. First, we must overcome our culturally conditioned beliefs and know with absolute certainty that outer biological approaches alone can never take us toward integral health and life. Without a more expansive consciousness that embraces the full scope and reach of the human experiences, narrow approaches such as conventional, alternative, and integrative medicines, with all their professionals, therapies, remedies, self-improvement programs, and psychological interventions, are merely detours.

The same can be said of the smorgasbord of the newest techniques, workshops, supplements, and seminars. I will not attempt to discourage you from trying these offerings. This is your right and perhaps the path you must first take. But unless you mature these experiences by simultaneously investing in a more comprehensive, inward-looking integral approach, these will become obstacles rather than resources.

If you overcome these obstacles, you will gradually shift your efforts toward an integral vision. The result will be a realignment of priorities, a growth of wisdom, an expansion of capacity, and a progressive unfolding of your unseen but ever-present innate potential for human flourishing.

THE THIRD POINT:
THE TRUTH OF THE INTEGRAL PATH

The integral path is holistic, evolutionary, intentional, person-centered, and dynamic. When we follow this path, it will invariably take us toward human flourishing.

The integral path affirms our innate wholeness. It does so by focusing on the four distinct yet interwoven aspects of our life: our psychospiritual, biological, interpersonal, and worldly life. Each aspect is part of the whole. As a result, it is not possible to heal any one aspect of our life or flourish into our full potential without attending to each of them. However, psychospiritual development drives the entire process. Without an expansive consciousness, we cannot fully evolve the other aspects of our life.

The integral path is an evolutionary path that views each aspect of our life as being in a state of evolution from body to mind to spirit, from outer to inner to innermost. Step-by-step, our body, mind, and spirit evolve to encompass a more comprehensive and accurate understanding of self and life, an enhanced capacity for health, and new and refined abilities. The integral path encourages and supports the attainment of our potential.

The integral path is intentional. Intention requires attention: the ability to voluntarily focus on a particular experience. Both of these mental faculties are uniquely interwoven in humankind. As a result, our approach to health becomes a conscious personal choice expressed through deliberate actions that are in accord with our intention. Integral health is neither imposed by culture nor required by life. We must choose and actualize it ourselves.

The integral path is person-centered. The individual is our primary concern. No two people have the same genetic makeup or life circumstance, manifest a disease in the same way, or sustain the same level of health. At any one moment, our movement toward integral health and life may require movement in any one or more of the four aspects of our life, with its lines and levels of development. Or perhaps the work of the moment is simply one of rest and regrouping. How can we who are practitioners know this unless we listen deeply to the other's whole story, commune in silence, and then allow an integral program to naturally arise? This approach appropriately honors the individual's uniqueness and right to be heard rather than seen through the generic lens of a specific approach or theory. We are not theories. Each of us is as unique as we are precious.

Finally, the integral approach is dynamic. It does not label you for life, forcing you and others to forever see you through this diagnostic fabrication. In the human condition, every moment is fresh and contains new possibilities. Where you were yesterday, you cannot possibly be tomorrow. As Heraclitus told us, it is impossible to step into the same stream twice. It may look like the same stream, but the water, the flow, the temperature, and everything else have changed.

The integral path correctly understands and appropriately responds to the character and possibilities of human life. That is what makes it a comprehensive, precise, and direct path to human flourishing

THE FOURTH POINT:
THE TRUTH OF THE FRUITS

The fruits of human flourishing—health, happiness, and wholeness—are the direct results of an integral approach to life.

Our daily life follows a simple, yet actually somewhat complex, pattern of cause and effect. At simple levels, this is quite apparent. For example, if we feel anger toward someone, they will invariably react to our anger. This is an immediate cause-and-effect relationship. In many aspects of life, including health, a number of factors must converge to create a sufficient cause for a later event. We can say with certainty that there are causes for suffering and causes for human flourishing. If we remove the causes of suffering, we will gain freedom from needless suffering, and if we create the causes of integral health, happiness, and wholeness, that is what we will get.

So, you might ask, how can this be done given the complexity of cause-and-effect equations? If we attempt to spend our life figuring out the subtleties of these relationships, it is certain that we will never figure them out before our death. Fortunately, we don't have to. Through a lifetime of intense dedication, the wise men and women from the past have sorted it out for us, and they are willing to share their wisdom with those who are ready to hear it.

Their advice is simple and consistent. *First,* become aware of and remove the causes of unnecessary suffering—the confusion, misunderstandings, and afflictions of the ordinary untrained mind. Stated another way, know what to cultivate in your life and what to abandon. Cultivate the understandings and actions that support integral health and abandon those that are obstacles and hindrances. *Next,* gradually train yourself to replace disturbing mental activity with loving-kindness. *Finally,* develop your consciousness through contemplative practice and your other capacities through a comprehensive program of integral practice. The result will be an inner calm, a discriminating and discerning wisdom, and an open heart. *These are the principal causes that give rise to human flourishing.* When we develop these innate qualities, sustained health, happiness, and wholeness will naturally follow. This step-by-step sequence of inner events leads from suffering to human flourishing. It's simply a matter of cause and effect. The wise ones have assured us of the certainty of this path.

The fruits will begin to emerge early in your work. We know from personal accounts and modern research that each step—our initial turn inward, our preparations, and our early efforts at practice—will lead to a noticeable, progressive enhancement of health, happiness, and wholeness. With time, your faith will be transformed into confidence, and with each passing day thereafter, your confidence will be further transformed until it becomes an unshakable certainty. Like a ripening fruit, you will not be able to reverse course. You will harvest the fruits of a well-lived life.

The entire process of integral assessment and practice will someday no longer be needed. That which informed, guided, supported, and sustained us will outlive its purpose. Then we will return to an ordinary life. But not the ordinary life we now live. It is a life that is fully aware, expansive, connected, open, loving, and quite simple. Each moment is filled with the delight of existence. Each interaction affirms the oneness of all. Each experience is unique and unrepeatable. Health is natural and easy. It is what we are when we are simply present in the magnificent mystery of life that is always and already within and without. In the end, we discover that a truly ordinary life *is* a precious life.

The
Fruits

Human Flourishing

14

Butter is the hidden sweet essence of milk. But for butter to emerge from milk, the milk must be churned. Health, happiness, and wholeness are similarly the unseen sweet essence of human life. To reveal this essence, we must develop ourselves and our life. As we have learned in this book, we can accomplish this by aspiring to a higher vision of health and engaging in integral practices that extend and expand our capacity and ability. In this way, we can evolve a new level of health that then gives rise to the unique treasures of human existence.

There are those, including the doubting voices within each of us, who will see this expansive vision as a fanciful and unrealizable utopian ideal. The habituated mind prefers to cling to familiar and limited ways of thinking about health and healing. But that is not what our times are about. In our deepest, most silent places, we each know that far more is possible than we have ever dreamt of. At this time in human development, we are called to live a life of the highest meaning and purpose.

This is not a new call. It is an old one found in the East and the West and in every culture and age when visionaries have sought to explore the unique nature of human life. Today's wise ones insist that humans are still an unfinished project, a work in progress. They seek to elevate human life by urging us toward perfection of our essential nature. They tell us that sustained health, happiness, and wholeness are natural to the human condition, but natural, they caution, does not mean immediately available. Go beyond human instincts that are stubborn holdovers from the animal kingdom. Look within at your humanity. You are not an animal disguised as a human. Unfold your nature. Become what a human is capable of becoming. Flourish.

This robust vision of the human possibility is consistently articulated, most often in mystery schools, over time and across cultures. All such visions have two common elements: a view of human life that celebrates humanity's unique potential and a road map that details the path to this highest quality of life. The integral approach to health is such an approach. It differs from all current approaches to health and healing because it fully addresses and encompasses all the unique possibilities of human life.

The integral approach asserts that each of us can choose to cultivate the best and highest human qualities and abilities. From this perspective, the fruits of human flourishing—authentic and sustained health, happiness, and wholeness—are the result of personal choice. As we choose to carefully and precisely cultivate what we are given, these three fruits emerge based on our level of development.

Integral practice leads to expanded consciousness. Expanded consciousness leads to a subtle mind. A subtle mind reveals our natural wisdom and loving-kindness. Wisdom and loving-kindness then unveil the human treasures we seek. This developmental sequence takes us from vision to practice to attainment. As we will discuss below, these qualities first arise in their most basic *outer* aspect, then in a more subtle *inner* aspect, and finally in their purest *innermost* essence. Each step and each unfolding expand our life and bring us closer to our fullest potential.

WHOLENESS

Let's start with wholeness and work our way through happiness to health. Wholeness is embedded in our very nature, so it cannot be stained, erased, or permanently obscured by disturbing emotions or an overactive conceptual mind. Our innate wholeness cannot be separated from our essence any more than water can be separated from wetness. Underneath all these veils, our original face—our wholeness—remains fresh and alive, awaiting our homecoming.

The first aspect of wholeness is its *outer* aspect, psychological wholeness. With personal effort and the help of a skilled guide, our unconscious and harmful habits and emotional reactions are diminished. We come to understand our mental afflictions, confusion, and doubts in terms of their childhood origins. New capacities are developed, our outer life is more balanced and satisfying, and we feel a growing sense of coherence and direction. Psychological development allows us to be in the world with less suffering, more freedom of choice, and far greater skill. It enhances our interpersonal relationships, matures our worldly activities, and decreases stress. With psychological development, we attain the outer level of wholeness.

We cannot leapfrog the outer aspect of wholeness in an attempt to go directly to the inner and innermost aspects. Psychological wholeness is a critical first step that takes time to properly unfold. It is important that we neither overestimate nor underestimate the importance and richness of this initial level of wholeness. In the first instance, we may overestimate the joy and ease gained from a healthy psychology, mistaking it for all that is possible. In the second instance, we may underestimate the importance of laying a proper foundation for further development. In either case, we may unknowingly stop at the outermost level.

The second aspect of wholeness is *inner* wholeness. We are no longer dealing with the content of our personality. We shift direction so our subtle inner life becomes our primary focus. Ongoing contemplative practice enables us to observe and study our moving mind, allowing us to tame and gain control over its ceaseless chatter. Step-by-step, we become capable of stabilizing clarity and stillness. Gradually, we experience the development of inner wholeness. It feels spacious, calm, stable, secure, easeful, and effortless. We feel more connected to ourselves and to others and less dependent on psychological understandings and strategies. Our sense of wholeness is far less subject to outer circumstances and mental movements.

Finally, we are ready for the fully ripened fruit of *innermost* wholeness. For this, we need to further expand our consciousness to experience the pure, pristine awareness of the subtlest mind. Our center is now located in existence itself, in the pure awareness that is the background upon which our mental activity floats. There is no separation in pure awareness. There is no I in pure awareness. Life *is* and we *are*—a seamless existence, an uninterrupted oneness, a perfect wholeness. However, only the unusual individual is able to stabilize this perfected wholeness. The rest of us need to see this final level as an ideal that beckons us.

Each time we touch a higher level of wholeness, we never return quite the same. We remember what it is to be more fully alive, what it feels like to be embedded in an immeasurable mystery. Instead of experiencing life through our thoughts and ideas about life, we experience life directly. To be fully whole is to be fully alive. This is the nature of the innermost, fully perfected wholeness.

HAPPINESS

Happiness is a uniquely human capacity. Animals are not capable of intentionally cultivating their outer behavior or developing their inner life. They are capable of moments of pleasure and satiation, but not of a sustained and conscious happiness. Humans alone can attain this extraordinary gift.

Because it is possible, all human beings seek happiness. But I'm not referring to the material or emotional pleasures of everyday life that we mistake as happiness. I'm referring to the authentic happiness that develops over time and in stages as we cultivate an inner life. Once experienced, genuine happiness permeates all aspects of our existence, flowing into our interpersonal relationships, balancing our physiology, and inspiring our worldly activities. Rather than reaching out to take pleasure from the world, we give happiness to the world from an inner, ever-replenished wellspring.

The *outer* aspect of happiness, as with wholeness, arrives with the development of a healthy personality. Psychological development allows us to discover the unconscious patterns that feed destructive emotions and their outer expression. As we uncover these patterns, diminish their influence in our life, and gradually replace them with loving-kindness, we progressively shift from a conflicted and unhealthy personality to a healthy one. We become skillful in our choices and in our actions. Our life takes a turn for the better. As a result, we begin to experience happiness in our relationships, work, and daily activities. This is an outer happiness.

A healthy personality and stabilized outer happiness become the foundation for *inner* happiness. Contemplative practice promotes a healthy and robust inner life. As a result, we feel calm, peaceful, and content with life as it is. We live more inside than outside, and many of our previously cherished outer experiences begin to fade in importance. We are happy just being in the stillness and spaciousness of the subtle mind. We slowly discover a special secret. The greatest pleasure we can have is experiencing a stable inner life. This inner happiness, for the first time, allows us to experience all of life's outer pleasures with joy and delight rather than craving, attachment, and suffering. This accomplishment brings a further stability and ripening of happiness.

Finally, as we touch the pure and pristine awareness of the subtlest mind, we discover *innermost* happiness. It is as if we have searched forever and finally found our beloved. Imagine the joy and exhilaration. But this is our inner Beloved. This is the One who has always been with us, awaiting the knock on the door of our innermost life. Here in silence, spaciousness, and clear awareness, we are united with our essence, our soul, our spirit—with existence itself. This subtle innerness gives us a profound and hardy happiness. The larger we grow our inner life, the more abundant this happiness will be. We have discovered an ever-replenishing wellspring of happiness. We are now able to fill the world with happiness, rather than grasp at it for fleeting pleasure.

HEALTH

Just as gold slowly reveals itself to the skilled craftsman who chips away at the outer stone, fully integrated, far-reaching integral health reveals itself to an integral practitioner who properly cultivates his or her life. Both inner and outer at the same time, this expansive health and well-being does not resemble what we now call health. We are not able to measure it with our machines or our laboratory tests. However intangible it may seem at first, we will know it with certainty when we experience it. All who are around us will similarly know it by the look on our face, the peace in our demeanor, and the energy we exude.

Our initial focus is on *outer* physical health, and this is important. We have learned to respond to the signs and symptoms of dysfunction or disease, visit a practitioner, undergo an assessment, and apply ourselves to a course of therapy. Maybe we have extended this to include prevention and promotion strategies that emphasize the importance of nutrition, fitness, and relaxation techniques. A healthy body is important, but it is only the first step on the path to integral health. Two other steps are needed.

The second level of health requires a second education, an *inner* education. To move toward this level of health, we must begin to transform our life from the inside out. With time and contemplative practice our reactive psychology changes into an inner stillness, dependent relationships are transformed into authentic intimacy, a stressful outer life gives way to a life of meaning and purpose, and focus on the anatomical body ripens into a focus on the subtle mind/body. This is a movement from outer regulation and outer health to self-regulation and inner health.

How does this shift to inner health feel? Our health is no longer exclusively defined by our body's physical capacity or a laboratory value. Well-being is far more than the presence or absence of physical health. We gain confidence in our ability to sustain this broader well-being through life's adversities, including disease, aging, and even death. We can now cultivate health on the inside. A newfound ease, freedom, and stability emerge with this deeper, more comprehensive experience of health.

Finally, we arrive at the *innermost,* or ultimate, aspect of health that is independent of the condition of our body. It is permanent and unchanging. Innermost health develops in tandem with a fully realized wholeness and happiness. What is so strange about this perfection of health is that it actually feels quite simple and ordinary. I'm here, we are all connected, and all is at ease precisely as it has always been and always will be. The only thing to do is to live, experience, and use what we have gained to serve others. This is the perfected flourishing of health.

As we progress toward integral health, there are many other gifts that we will gather along the way. We will evolve the mental abilities of clarity, attention, intention, visualization, memory recall, creative imagination, and extended perceptual skills. We will deepen our empathy, sensitivity, compassion, courage, patience, perseverance, resilience, and capacity for intimacy and universal loving-kindness. Our body may gain in strength, flexibility, agility, and endurance. The most subtle forms of self-regulation become possible. Integral development evolves so that we realize our fullest potential.

A TASTE OF HUMAN FLOURISHING

Although fully developed and sustained levels of health, happiness, and wholeness can only emerge through a progressive process of inner development, we can each experience a taste of these possibilities. Why is this possible? It is possible because the essence of human flourishing is already and always within us. It is merely obscured from view. Like the sun breaking through the clouds, it can become visible and experienced briefly prior to its full development, only to be covered up once again. These tastes can in themselves accelerate the developmental process by intensifying our motivation, familiarizing us with our final goal, and catalyzing our practices.

By practicing the following creative visualization, you can experience a taste of human flourishing. Find a quiet time of the day and allot thirty minutes for this practice. Begin by finding a comfortable place, sit in a chair or on a cushion, and relax into the ease and peace of your undisturbed mind and body. There is no need to begin a formal practice session. Just rest quietly and follow the guided visualization. You might find it easiest to record this practice onto an audiotape by reading the text aloud and pausing at the appropriate places, or you can obtain a recording of these practices (see the Resource Guide).

With your eyes closed, bring to mind a time of great happiness. Perhaps there is a special place, person, or experience that most reminds you of this. Invite this experience into the present moment and allow it to fully saturate your awareness. If you cannot recall such an experience, then use your imagination to create one as you might imagine it would be. Allow this feeling of great happiness to unfold in all its details and to penetrate your whole being.

What does it look like? How does your body feel? Are there any sounds or special smells? What is the quality of your mind? What is your sense of self? Are you feeling a sense of spaciousness, harmony, and connectedness? How does your spirit feel? Allow this experience to intensify as if you were turning up a water spigot. Pause here for a while and fully enjoy this taste of happiness.

Next, bring to mind a time in which you experienced a sense of wholeness, oneness, connection, and flow. Invite it into the present moment and allow it to fully saturate your awareness. Perhaps it was a moment of love, personal achievement, athletic activity, or immersion in nature. If you cannot recall such an image, use your imagination to create one. Allow this image and the feeling flowing from it to unfold in all its details and to penetrate your whole being.

What does it look like? How does your body feel? Are there any sounds or special smells? What is the quality of your mind? What is your sense of self? Are you feeling a sense of spaciousness, harmony, and connectedness? How does your spirit feel? Allow this experience to intensify as if you were turning up a water spigot. Pause here for a while and fully enjoy this taste of wholeness.

Finally, bring to mind a time you experienced exuberant vitality, radiant health, and well-being. Recall a time when you felt filled with energy and life. Invite this image and felt sense into the present moment and allow it to fully saturate your aware-ness. Perhaps it was a moment of love, personal achievement, athletic activity, or an immersion in nature. If you cannot recall such an image, use your imagination to cre-ate one as you might imagine it would be. Allow this image to unfold in all its details and to penetrate your whole being.

What does it look like? How does your body feel? Are there any sounds or special smells? What is the quality of your mind? What is your sense of self? Are you feeling a sense of spaciousness, harmony, and connectedness? How does your spirit feel? Allow this experience to intensify as if you were turning up a water spigot. Pause here for a while and fully enjoy this taste of radiant health.

Allow these three experiences to merge together so that health, happiness, and wholeness become a single experience. Fully enjoy this essence of your being. Know that it arises within you. Your outer circumstances are unchanged and you have neither been medicated nor otherwise manipulated. This is your natural essence and being that is always and already within you. How does the quality of this innerness affect what you bring to others and the world? What obscures this essence? Why have you left this home? Remain with this experience for the remainder of the session.

After the session, observe how this inner and innermost experience flows into your daily life. Similarly, observe the veils that appear and slowly begin to obscure the full experience of health, happiness, and wholeness. What are these veils? Are they thoughts, emotions, or busyness? Can you see how the habitual patterns of your mind and life take over? Recognize that the obstacles that separate you from a life of sus-tained human flourishing can be overcome with commitment and practice. Allow this taste of health, happiness, and wholeness to motivate your practice. What is more important than the treasures of integral health and life?

In Chapter 1, I told you the story of an old fisherman who went down to the sea each morning before dawn. One morning he found a little pouch filled with what he thought were stones and began throwing them one at a time into the sea. When dawn broke, he had one left, and to his shock, he discovered it was a diamond. He had tossed all the other gems into the ocean. We don't have to do that.

Even though it may be a bit difficult to see these gems of human life through the limited vision of our culture, we can trust the wise teachers and our intuition that there is more to life than we have imagined. With faith, we can open our mind and heart and take the courageous first steps on the path to integral health. Ultimately, this choice will bring the most profound meaning to our existence and crown our life with the precious gems of human flourishing—health, happiness, and wholeness.

The Center for
Human Flourishing

15

If you or I needed physical healing today, we would know exactly where to go and what to do. But if we wanted integral health, we wouldn't know where to turn. If we had ample resources, we might spend a weekend or week at a spa. In addition to being pampered, we would be offered a variety of opportunities that might range from massage to yoga, cooking classes, or relaxation techniques. Or we could attend a program at a spiritual center, focusing on our inner life. But where would we go for the guidance and support needed for a fully integrated and far-reaching integral approach? Where would we go to embrace a new and expansive vision of our possibilities, to find skillful and committed integral practitioners, and to share our journey with a like-minded community?

For more than 800 years, the Aesclepian healing temples served these purposes given the resources and skill of the Greek culture at that time. There were hundreds of such centers to choose from. However, this is not the case today, and that absence cannot be filled by conventional medical centers, integrative-care programs, spas, or spiritual centers. Healing centers that currently focus on integrating alternative and complementary approaches extend the outer approaches of biomedical centers, but they do not fundamentally alter them. While they have added to our medical toolbox and here and there flirted with other aspects of being, they have mostly missed the broader intent of an integral approach. Each makes its own contribution, but none is integral in scope.

If humanity is to evolve to integral health, it is imperative to create a healthcare system that encourages and supports our efforts. We also need a community of trained professionals and like-minded friends who support our efforts. We cannot do this work alone in an unsympathetic culture. We need a safe haven in which to develop sufficient inner stability to allow us to do meaningful work in the outer world without being constantly pulled away from our inner life. An entirely new, more broad-based healing center is needed to nurture and promote the five principles of integral healing. We call this The Center for Human Flourishing. This healing center needs to embody the integral vision and be staffed by healers who have walked this path so that center will have the scope and depth needed to accomplish its ambitious mission—helping humanity take the evolutionary step to integral health.

As individuals, as a culture, and as a global village, we must expand our limited and limiting vision of health. In order to unfold the fullness of our personal potential and live cooperatively and successfully in a very complex world, we need integral health rather than partial health. Only then can we carefully use our sophisticated technologies to address the challenges of multiculturalism, and bring worldwide poverty and the many heart-wrenching problems created by it to an end. We must exceed the limits of our current consciousness because wisdom and compassion are needed more desperately now than ever. For the world to become a truly healthy global village, we need to avail ourselves of the full gifts of our humanity.

Years ago, in an effort to understand how such a cultural shift could occur, I studied the process by which our current system of scientific medicine came into existence. I wanted to know exactly how we succeeded in replacing an entrenched and outdated system of eclectic practitioners and their apprentice-style education. So I traveled from archive to archive in this country to study the transformation in medicine that occurred during the brief fifty years from 1870 to 1920. What I discovered was rather astonishing.

There were only three basic requirements for change. The first and most essential was a vision of change whose time had come. The second was a few forward-looking, pivotal individuals who could see the future of medicine and were willing to steadfastly promote it against the prevailing and entrenched interests of the time. The final element was philanthropic support for the initial demonstration project and the effort needed to extend this approach to the entire culture. Once this vision caught on, it spread rapidly.

We can take hope from this history lesson. Now we know fundamental change requires a vision whose time has come, devoted, far-seeing leadership, and a demonstration project supported by philanthropic or public funding. The time is ripe for the realization of the integral vision. What would a Center for Human Flourishing look like? How would people use it? Let's imagine what is needed to make this a reality.

THE BLUEPRINT FOR
A CENTER FOR HUMAN FLOURISHING

Let's begin the blueprint for such a center by examining the integral vision and the integral map. From there, we'll look at the setting for the center, its appearance and ambience, the characteristics of practitioners, the activities of the center, and its extension into the community.

The Vision

The mission of the center is to alleviate suffering and to promote human flourishing—integral health, happiness, and wholeness—first for ourselves and then for others. The activities of the center will address the full range of human experience—psychospiritual, biological, interpersonal, and worldly. Each individual who visits the center needs to have a clear understanding of the integral vision and map, though that may be no more than a vague familiarity for the first-time visitor. The ideal place for a retreat facility is in proximity to an urban center.

Why a retreat center? Each person must have a regular opportunity to extract his or her self from daily life with its many demanding activities and distractions. We can then fully focus on the steps involved in turning ourselves toward human flourishing. In a sense, this may seem indulgent. But in actuality, it is required to create integral health and life. Consider the fact that when we become ill, we are forced to drop everything and spend whatever time is necessary to regain our health. This is usually outer health alone. Do we have to be sick in order to find time for our health? Do we have to be sick in order to give ourselves permission to invest in integral health and life?

There are three levels of retreat: outer, inner, and innermost. Each will be available at the center. Each of these is important. The outer retreat is an external environment of stillness and solitude free from the normal activities and distractions of daily life. This outer environment supports the inner and innermost aspects of retreat. The inner aspect is not located in a physical location. It is in the mind. So it may take time to develop. We enter an inner retreat when our mind is emptied of its usual distractions, centered in stillness, and infused with loving-kindness. The inner retreat allows time, space, and quiet needed for contemplative practices that support integral health. In time, the inner retreat will give way to the innermost retreat. This occurs when we touch the subtlest mind and its pristine awareness and precise and penetrating wisdom.

The retreat setting will be a sanctuary, a sacred place where we can attend to our life with care and devotion. It will be a place of physical beauty that encompasses both the natural and the built environment. It will mirror back to us the solitude and harmony we seek to discover in all aspects of our life. The center and its environs will feel like our natural home, reflecting the ease, peace, and embrace that lie within. Every detail will be uplifting, supportive, and conducive to integral practice and personal development.

The Healers

Each member of the staff will be a healer in his or her own way. This includes the individual who answers the telephone, kitchen helpers, and the cleaning and support staff. The integral process will be the foremost aim of everyone involved in all the center's activities. That will allow a healing presence to be felt through a gentle word, a thoughtful gesture, a kind touch, or a listening ear. That can serve as both reassurance and an example of what should be possible in all human interactions.

The healing practitioner will be central to the center's activities. Each practitioner will be involved in his or her ongoing integral transformative process. To model and teach this special work requires not merely book learning, but direct hands-on instruction in the many practices that facilitate the path to human flourishing. Practitioners will be involved in this sacred work because it is of prime importance in their own life. For them, helping others to similarly find their way is part of their own integral process. In a sense, these individuals are the Aesclepians of the modern-day healing center, catalyzing the healing process while simultaneously helping to build the personal skills and capacities of others. Their intention is to assist each individual in developing mastery of the integral process and assuming his or her rightful role as self-healer as soon as possible.

These practitioners will be different from the technically oriented practitioners we are familiar with. Their background and training will be varied. But what they share and emphasize in their work is knowledge of the integral path and fluency with integral practice. They are generalists in the integral path while they may also be specialists in one particular modality.

The Healing Relationship

The practitioner's knowledge will be complemented by his or her skillful capacity to listen with full attention. This special type of listening will serve two purposes. To begin, one listens with a contemplative mind and a clear, unbiased awareness. This is accompanied by the intention to fully hear the other regardless of the time involved. In this way, the healer is entrained or drawn into the other's experience. So the practitioner becomes fully empathic and fully aware of the circumstances of the individual's life. As a result, both the practitioner and the individual are able to arrive at a clear sense of the next step toward integral health. Together, they will determine what aspect or aspects of the individual's life are ready to be worked with and what practices would suit this individual.

The second aspect of the listening process is what we will call "reverse entrainment." As the practitioner takes on the life experience of the individual, the individual simultaneously takes on the contemplative state of the practitioner. When this occurs, the practitioner can point out the nature and character of the subtle mind experienced by the individual. This is an essential first introduction to the inner life, which unfolds naturally from the listening process. From there, inner practice can be more fully developed.

The meeting of the practitioner and the individual thus serves as both an ongoing assessment process and a healing process. The bond formed here will be a long-term relationship. The healer remains available until the individual has developed the capacities and resources to assume full responsibility for self-healing. Clearly, we are not referring to a childlike dependent relationship. Here the intent of the practitioner is to liberate the individual from the need for any healer except the one inside. He or she accomplishes that by providing the appropriate vision, skills, understanding, encouragement, and support.

Having arrived at a full assessment, the practitioner and individual develop an integral plan tailored to the unique needs of the individual and involving one or more of the four aspects of life—psychospiritual, biological, interpersonal, and worldly. This plan, accompanied by the proper resources to sustain it, becomes the starting point in a dynamic process that aids in the recovery from disease or distress and promotes integral health and well-being. This process will continue day after day until the individual is ready to return home. The entire process will occur in the context of a supportive community of like-minded individuals.

Integral Practice

The healing center will be designed like a wheel with a hub and its spokes. The hub is the ongoing relationship between the practitioner and the individual. It is the center of the integral approach. From this core relationship specific activities and practices radiate outward like the spokes of a wheel. The focus and particular resources of the heal-ing plan will vary according to the needs of the individual, but they will steadfastly be aimed in the direction of human flourishing.

With increasing facility in contemplative practice, the individual will slowly, at his or her own pace, shift the center of healing from the outside—the center and its resources—to the inside—his or her consciousness and its resources. Simultaneously, the relationship with the practitioner will also undergo change as the individual pro-gressively takes on the role of self-healer. This is the step that never occurred at the Aesclepian healing centers. There, the healer always remained outside in the form of Asclepius. In our time and in such a center, it is the clear intent of integral practice that the individual takes back the powers previously attributed to a god. Human beings are now capable of this essential shift.

Returning Home

Retreats always come to an end. They are not meant to be permanent, but rather a special space in time to allow us to focus without distraction on our life. They are meant as a preparation for worldly life rather than as a substitute or antidote for it. Although the individual may leave the center, the center will not leave the individual. The entire experience—the relationships, personal growth, practices, and other resources—will become part of the individual's life. Of even greater importance, the vision of human flourishing, the knowledge of what is now possible, and the hopeful-ness and confidence that have been attained will endure in the heart and mind of each person who experiences the center and its staff. The center will remain a home to return to again and again until that home is firmly and securely situated in the spirit and soul of all who undertake this process.

Returning to the everyday home will bring challenges, so the proper preparations must be made. An ongoing set of practices, study, reading materials, and sustained con-tact with the center and its extended community will assist in this transition. In time, there will be little difference between a retreat and worldly life. This is, in fact, the aim. We seek to bring healing into our life each day and to transform our daily life into a healing environment. We learn to use life's offerings and challenges as teachers and teachings. This, as you remember from Chapter 12, was the second aspect of inte-gral practice—using life as a practice.

Each of us who leaves a retreat should be encouraged to write a testimonial such as those written by people leaving Aesclepian healing temples. Encouraged by a community that will support our efforts, we should experience a previously unknown aliveness, enhanced capacity for health, new and expanded abilities, and steadfast confidence in our ability to continue our movement toward integral health and life.

JOURNEY TO THE CENTER FOR HUMAN FLOURISHING

Close your eyes for a moment and imagine taking the same trip that the ancient Greeks did on their way to the Aesclepian healing temple. You know—perhaps through suffering, illness, or the calling of your soul—that you are ready to turn a corner in your life. Fortunately, there is a place to go for individuals seeking integral health and life. You call such a center and are warmly received and encouraged to visit. On your way, your thoughts about daily life and its routines drop away, and your focus slowly turns toward your own life. You feel a mixture of hope and excitement tempered with apprehension.

You arrive at the center, and you feel at home in the natural beauty as stillness and warmth welcome you. You meet the staff, find your room, get settled in, and sit back and read a bit about the center, its mission, and its activities. You then join other new guests to learn more about what lies ahead. At this initial meeting, several practitioners serve as guides. They introduce themselves one at a time, speaking about their life, work, and interests. With whom do you feel a sense of connection or initial chemistry? Perhaps this is the first practitioner you will interview. Is he or she a match for your needs? Chemistry and intimacy are essential for this process to truly work.

Imagine meeting with this healer/helper. Imagine your story is fully heard from beginning to end, acknowledged, understood, and embraced. Experience the sense of stillness that enters your mind and heart. How does it feel to experience this inner stillness, peace, and ease? Your practitioner will point out that this is your inner healer, your place of refuge and reliance. Sitting in communion, imagine how you and your mentor will slowly arrive at the direction to take and the resources and activities to explore in your healing.

Each day you engage in activities that nourish your body, mind, and spirit. Gradually, you begin to gain new understandings that blossom into important realizations. You can now sense how it is possible to change from the inside out. Your faith is transformed into confidence. You feel early movement toward integral health.

You can now trust there is a place and a way to find what you have been seeking. You now know that integral health and life is available to you regardless of your circumstances. Health, happiness, and wholeness can be self-cultivated, grown, and continuously expanded. Nothing and nobody can permanently separate you from these innate but previously elusive treasures. It is your natural state untainted and untouched by life's adversities. You feel release and great relief.

There will come a time when you will be ready to return to worldly life. You will be renewed and encouraged by your experience at the center. You will have gained an understanding of the integral vision, acquired a program of integral practice, and discovered an inner path. This integral path can now become your new retreat and refuge, your source of reliance. You will return home connected to the new community met at the retreat and to the center that will always be a home away from home.

Things will be a bit different when you return home. You will have new priorities and perhaps have to make some readjustments. You will need solitude and time for study and reflection. You will soon notice that you will be less reactive to life's challenges and have more patience and an increasingly clear sense of direction. You will certainly sense the awakening of a newfound health, happiness, and wholeness. This is the vision of healing bequeathed to us by the great sages. How does this feel to you? Would you like this to be more than an imaginary journey? Let's make it happen.

This chapter provided a brief overview of a new and very different type of healing center that will serve as a resource for individuals—adults and children—a teaching center for practitioners-in-training, and a research center for those who wish to more deeply study this expansive healing process. Everything we need to create such a center is waiting and ready. All that is needed is to implement the vision we have described here. Now is the time to bring it to life. To do so will be an act of healing not just for ourselves but our culture and the whole world.

Life Divine

16

If human life is endowed with a spark of the divine, it would most certainly reveal itself as the highest and best in us. There can be little doubt that our highest and best is our capacity for self-reflection, penetrating wisdom, and universal loving-kindness. If we choose to ripen these qualities, their essence will flow into each aspect of our life, bringing about a gradual perfection of health, happiness, and wholeness.

We cannot expect this to be the direction or intention of the popular mass culture as that rarely aspires to the highest and the best. So you and I are key to this integral movement, for it is we alone who can choose to fully develop our consciousness and our life. If we are to flourish as individuals, we must see it as *our* direction and manifest it as *our* intention. We must take charge and guide our evolution from body to mind to spirit. Only the integral process will uncover our divine spark that now is concealed by our focus on the physical and obscured by an overactive mental life but will finally be revealed through spiritual development.

OUR TIME IS NOW

Some would say we should go slowly—just a little bit at a time. Or as the poet T. S. Eliot put it, " . . . humans cannot bare much of reality." There is great truth in this observation. Yet, at the same time, there is paradoxically within each of us an innate and relentless longing for this greater reality, for this larger, more perfected life. To settle for less, to be satisfied with merely improving our health and our life is to ignore this deepest reality and most profound aspect of our humanity. That is why it is essential to explore the subtle mind, enhance our capacity, extend our abilities, and seek human flourishing rather than dumbing integral health down to an assortment of relaxation techniques, self-improvement programs, psychological understandings, or more remedies and therapies.

It might have been easier to write another "7-day program." But this is not the truth of our human capacities. The truth is that we have been blessed with profound intellectual and spiritual abilities and to water down this human potential for practical or commercial reasons is a foolishness that we and our world can no longer afford. Our world is too complex for simple answers that will fail to further our personal and shared life. I am certain that we can digest the truth we yearn for. It is now time to look toward the genius of human life.

Integral development is the way we uncover this genius. It is the only antidote for a troubled life and a troubled world. When we engage an integral process, the work we do inside is the work that the world so urgently needs. Where there is inner peace, there is outer peace. Where there is inner harmony, there is outer harmony. Where there is inner health, there is outer health. Healing ourselves is healing others. An integral life begets an integral world. In this way, we become the doctor, the nurse, and the medicine to ourselves and to the larger community of humankind.

ADDRESSING THE GAP

As I write this final chapter, I am painfully aware of the gap between this lofty vision and the reality of our life and our world. Biological imperatives still have the power to pull us back to preoccupation with survival and physical needs. Psychological conditioning can easily force us to live more instinctually than intentionally. It is difficult to clear a new path. Yet, here and there, we must remember to take a deep breath and to focus inward in order to remember who we really are, why I am compelled to write this book, and you to read it.

This recognition of the gap between what we aspire to and what actually is can serve to motivate us. A certain strength and determination will not give in to the forces of darkness and conformity. There is too much at stake. So we study, practice, go on retreat, pursue integral health, and gradually come to know that life *can* be transformed. In so doing, we become more confident that these efforts make a difference and that it is our responsibility to promote and pursue this noble path.

It is now important to return to where we started. I began this book by discussing the preciousness of human life and the possibility of gaining freedom from suffering for ourselves and others through a flourishing of body, mind, and spirit. Now we know how to move in that direction. It is for each of us to choose in our deepest silence whether we wish to take this adventure of a lifetime. The poet Christopher Fry said it the following way:

Dark and cold we may be, but this
Is no winter now. The frozen misery
Of centuries breaks, cracks, begins to move,
The Thunder is the thunder of the floes,
The thaw, the flood, the upstart Spring,
Thank God our time is now when wrong
Comes up to face us everywhere,
Never to leave us till we take
The longest stride of soul men ever took.
Affairs are now soul size
The enterprise
Is exploration into God.
Where are you making for? It takes
So many thousand years to wake,
But will you wake for pity's sake?

We are finally awakening to the ageless longing of our soul. Now more than ever, we can hear its call to fulfill a destiny that has long been encoded in our heart. We are ripe for transformation. Our time is now—irrespective of all that comes up to meet us. Our time is now, right now, this moment, and there is no time to waste. Are we ready to awake? What awaits us is no less than a profound and enduring health, happiness, and wholeness. That is the genius, and culmination of a perfected human life. That's the essence of a life divine.

All shall be captured by delight, transformed:
In waves of undreamed ecstasy shall roll
Our mind and life and sense and laugh in a light
Other than this hard limited human day,
The body's tissues thrill apotheosised,
Its cells sustain bright metamorphosis.

—SRI AUROBINDO

The Evolution
of Medicine

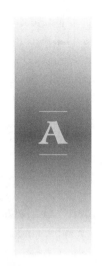

Humankind has been on a perpetual quest to improve and enhance health. The ongoing development of medicine has led to the progressive expansion of our vision of health and approach to healing. Change has occurred over extended periods of time resulting in a medicine of greater complexity, capacity, and comprehensiveness. Each evolutionary leap has embraced all previous approaches and transcended their limitations.

From our initial preoccupation with survival to our modern medical science to our current efforts at prevention and health promotion, we have responded to the challenges and opportunities of the time to evolve more capable medicine. From the perspective of any one time in history, it is often difficult to see this larger landscape of change. Yet without this broader view we are unable to see that medicine is and has always been evolving.

Our current approach to medicine emerged as a response to the failure of previous levels of medicine to control infectious epidemics of years past. The achievements of medical science have largely resolved this challenge to human life, but its success has highlighted a new set of challenges. As a result, we are now facing previously unknown epidemics of mental distress and premature degenerative disease. In attempting to deal with these modern-day epidemics, modern medicine has reached its limits. Our challenge today is to comprehensively and innovatively address and heal these causes of suffering, which diminish the quality of life and hinder progress toward human flourishing.

This challenge presents itself as an evolutionary crisis, a pivotal point in which we grow as a species into a larger humanity or stagnate in the past. This evolutionary crisis is seen most clearly in medicine. Our choice is to remain exclusively fixated on our biological health or to take the next leap in our evolution toward a comprehensive and far-reaching integral health—what we have also called ultimate health. The first requires no more than an expansion of our existing medical tool kit. The second requires that we emphatically say yes to human life and its extraordinary possibilities. This requires that we resolve our evolutionary crisis in health and healing through a leap in consciousness that transcends our limited and conventional notions of health and liberates these higher possibilities.

EXPANSION AND TRANSFORMATION

There are two approaches to change—expansion and transformation. Our efforts to address modern-day epidemics must consider both. In Figure A, the inner circles reflect expansion and the outer arrows reflect transformation. Expansion seeks to extend the scope and reach of the current medical model. It increases the size of the medical tool kit. It is horizontal in direction. Transformation is evolutionary, developmental, and vertical in direction. It leaps to a more encompassing vision that transcends the limitations of the current model while embracing its achievements.

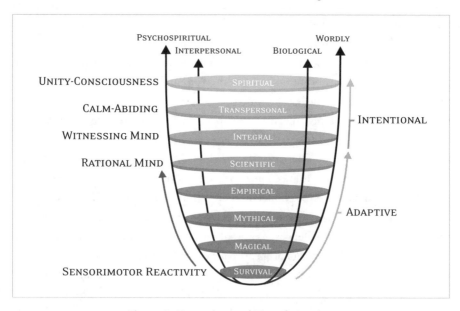

Figure A. Expansion and Transformation

With few exceptions our current approaches—conventional, alternative, energetic, and integrative—are limited to biological and physical interventions, or at best

reach out to touch the other aspects of human life. But these approaches are not transformative. They expand but do not fundamentally alter the existing model. The integral approach asserts these two dimensions of change. It is holistic in that it reaches out
to all aspects of the human experience and transformational in its upward evolutionary
movement from body to mind to spirit.

Figure A highlights the evolutionary development of medicine from its origins in
survival to its culmination in spiritual medicine. We will explore several important
features of this diagram.

1. Each leap in medicine is associated with a corresponding leap in consciousness. In
   fact, it is the expansion of consciousness that actually drives the transformation of
   medicine.

2. From the earliest survival "medicine" to present-day medical science, people have
   reacted to the contemporary challenges to health. This is a *reactive* approach to
   health that is driven by fear. All future efforts will be *intentional*. Rather than reacting to a health threat, we will be choosing integral health.

3. Each shaded disk represents an historical approach to health and healing. Through
   the efforts of its adherents, this approach is expanded and perfected within the
   bounds of its initial vision. The vertical evolutionary leap to the next level of
   medicine is a radical shift in vision that embraces all preceding approaches while
   transcending their limitations. We fill in this new approach through horizontal
   expansion. As this approach reaches its full maturity, we again see a series of new
   initiatives designed to address its increasingly apparent limitations. Eventually, with
   a growth in consciousness and vision, we evolve to the next level of health. Horizontal expansion and vertical transformation are the two active components of
   evolution in medicine. They work together to advance our understanding and
   capacity for health.

4. Each approach to medicine, to one extent or another, considers the four aspects of
   the human experience. The four aspects are represented in Figure A by arrow-
   tipped lines. At the lower levels of development, there is a maximum attention to
   biological survival and less to the other aspects of life. This will shift as we move up
   the evolutionary ladder. As we successfully address the biological dilemmas of
   humankind, more attention will be given to previously neglected aspects of human
   experience. That is what is happening today. Our leap is to integral health.

5. You will notice that I have included two levels of health and healing that go beyond
   the integral approach. They rely on the most subtle levels of consciousness.

6. Evolution is a messy business. Although the general movement is ascent, there is some back and forth. A society threatened by great social disaster may descend to survival mode. An infectious epidemic will firmly plant us in scientific medicine. A well-functioning society will aim toward integral health and healing. The skills and capacities gained with each level of development can be called upon when needed. We are merely transcending the limitations of earlier approaches, not rejecting them.

THE MODERN-DAY EVOLUTION IN MEDICINE

When dealing with the limitations of contemporary medicine, a variety of attempts have been made to reform it. These changes have served to increase our therapeutic modalities, expand the scope of our efforts, and, finally, bring us toward authentic integral change. This is a gradual process, with the earlier horizontal initiatives preparing us for the vertical shift to integral health and healing.

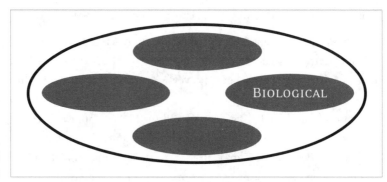

Figure B.
Biological
Health

Figure B depicts today's conventional medicine. The focus is exclusively on the biological aspect of life. The same emphasis is generally found in alternative, complementary, energetic, integrative, and what many call holistic medicine. Each of these contributes to an expansion and integration of approaches, remedies, therapies, and techniques. We have expanded the therapeutic modalities of medicine by increasing the size of the medical tool kit. But the biological focus has remained the same.

Figure C depicts the scope of a genuine holistic and integrative approach. Here, the terms "holistic" and "integration" refer to a concern with all aspects of the human experience. This is in distinction to the current use of the terms to indicate blending of multiple approaches, therapies, and remedies under a single umbrella. A genuine holistic approach respects the multidimensionality of the human experience and the interconnectedness between all aspects of our being.

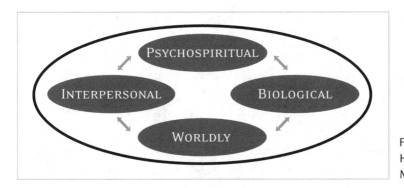

Figure C.
Holistic
Medicine

Authentic holism further expands the range and scope of health and healing by addressing the whole person and the practices that pertain to each aspect of an individual's life. In any approach—conventional, alternative, energetic, and integrative—there are outstanding practitioners who practice from this truly holistic perspective. However, as noted before, the majority of practitioners in their actual day-to-day practice remain within the bounds of the biological focus.

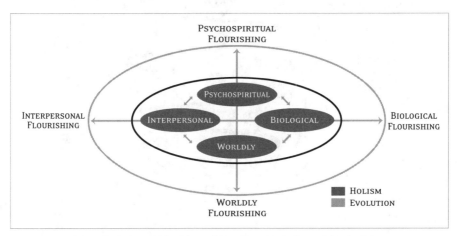

Figure D. Integral Health and Healing: Holistic and Evolutionary

Integral medicine is both holistic and evolutionary. Figure D depicts these two defining aspects. The inner oval designates and distinguishes the holistic aspect of the integral approach that addresses all aspects of the human experience, and the outer oval adds an evolutionary aspect that addresses growth and development. In actuality, they work together.

In Figures B through D, we can see a visual representation of our current and future approaches to health and healing. We can see the early efforts at reform that are largely expansionary, and the final evolutionary leap to integral medicine. Preparations are necessary for the final leap. But we cannot mistake them for the fully realized transformative change. The latter entirely shifts the vision, approach, practitioner, and practice of medicine.

THE EVOLUTIONARY SPIRAL

Medicine is continuously spiraling out in its evolutionary growth. But there is no guarantee here. It can only advance through our choices and actions. As a result, we are all responsible for this ongoing movement toward more expansive health and healing. We do our part by taking the next step in our own life toward integral health. In doing so, we prepare the ground for others and for further leaps in medicine.

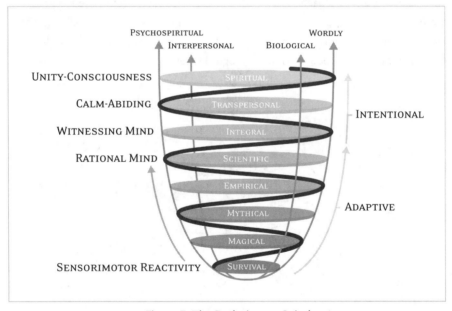

Figure E. The Evolutionary Spiral

Figure E depicts the outward spiraling of evolutionary change, the movement toward greater complexity and capacity. As the spiral comes to the end of an era, it begins to turn toward the next leap. This movement is prepared by expansionary change and completely by a transformational leap. The leap itself is a dramatic and permanent shift in consciousness, capacity, and vision. That's where we are today.

For the Practitioner

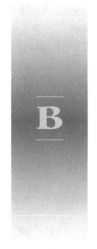

B

As medicine grows in understanding and capacity, practitioners must similarly evolve. In many instances, practitioners themselves will be the leading edge of change; in other instances, it is important for us to keep apace with change that is already in progress. In many respects this is not unlike our customary continuing education. It is an update and expansion of our existing knowledge and methods. We learn about the most recent research, new techniques, and emerging therapies.

The continuing education we discuss here is different. It is not horizontal in nature. It does not focus on expanding the current paradigm. It is transformative. This type of change occurs infrequently, yet when it does, it requires that we step up to a new vision, grow our consciousness, expand our capacity, and develop new skills and abilities. We are very fortunate that this is our current circumstance.

It is a special experience for me to be able to share this new and emerging approach with my fellow practitioners. It is special because I share with you a growing frustration with both our current approach to health and healing whose limitations are increasingly apparent and our efforts at reform that have failed to evolve medicine to an integral perspective. I also share with you the desire to practice a more comprehensive and meaningful approach to health and healing. And I share with you the desire to re-infuse soul and meaning into medicine for ourselves and for our patients.

In my personal and professional experience, I can assure you that I have found the integral approach to be precisely what we are looking for. It is practical, comprehensive, and well developed, and will take us to the next level of healing. However, it is not just a new remedy, technique, or therapy. It requires us to first bring an integral approach into our own lives. We are not just expanding the medical tool kit. We are transforming medicine and evolving it to a new level. That means the holder of the tool kit, the practitioner himself or herself, must enter the transformative process. We must change ourselves if we are to change the medicine we are practicing. I am sure you will find, as have I, that this is not a chore but a privilege and opportunity. It is what we have always sought—to be closer to the soul of healing and to develop ourselves into rich and talented healers.

THE CORE COMPONENTS OF AN INTEGRAL PRACTICE

There are seven essential aspects to an integral practice.

1. The Integral Map

2. The Healer

3. The Healee

4. The Integral Relationship

5. The Integral Diagnosis

6. The Integral Prescription

7. The Setting

1. The Integral Map

The *integral map* is the foundation of an integral practice. It outlines the principles that distinguish this approach from others. The integral map provides a truly holistic, fully integrated, and evolutionary approach to health. We use the word "integrative" here to refer to the process of integrating and addressing the four aspects of the human experience, not integrating a variety of methods, remedies, and therapies. What we seek to evolve is the full potential and capacity of each individual in each aspect of life. Our map is based on the five guiding principles: holistic, evolutionary, intentional, person-centered, and dynamic.

The aspiring integral practitioner should study two underlying aspects of this map: the backbone that relies on integral theory as elaborated by the contemporary philosopher Ken Wilber and its application to health and healing as elaborated in this book. Together, these two sources will offer a broad perspective on the integral process. Other suggested materials are provided in the Resources Guide.

2. The Healer

The healer is the key to the evolution and fulfillment of the integral healing process. This cannot be emphasized enough. In the Introduction, I referred to my second medical education in the East. This gave me the opportunity to develop fluency with the inner aspects of health and life. Without this education, it would not have been possible for me to go beyond my training. To become the agents of a more expansive health, we must begin with our own life. This is not only book learning. It is hands-on learning. This means that we must be willing to explore the inner aspects of our own life through psychological development and contemplative practice. This is the most undeveloped aspect of our life and of our current approaches to medicine. We must start with preparations and practice. Nothing less will do.

By incorporating the integral process into our own lives, I am certain that we will each discover the profound possibilities of integral health and healing. What begins as professional training soon becomes far more personal. We begin to know firsthand what can actually happen as we evolve a more expansive life. We come to know that the alleviation of suffering and the ascent to human flourishing are more than ideas. We can taste them ourselves. We gain confidence in this higher possibility. We want to end human suffering. Our personal work becomes a sacred responsibility, a way that we can help others and create a better world. Health and healing become alive for us. The soul of medicine returns.

3. The Healee

What I will say here applies to the healer as well as to the patient. In the East, there is a metaphor that tells us how to gauge the readiness of an individual to engage a new vision. They call it the "three pot" metaphor. An individual is not ready to leap to another understanding and level of health if he or she is like a pot turned upside down. This individual is not open to hear anything new so it is useless to share something of such great depth. An individual who is like a pot with a hole in the bottom will not be able to hold what is given to him or her. This person cannot absorb and remember the essence of what is taught. He or she is not ready for something new. A dirty pot cannot receive knowledge without coloring and distorting it with inaccurate interpretations. If one's beliefs are so fixed that they are not open to alternative views, then one is similarly not ready to evolve to a higher level of knowledge or capacity. Whether we are a healer or a patient, we must be ready to receive and consider the integral approach. If not, it should not be shared. We then meet the patient where he or she is within their belief system. We build trust and wait for an opening. It is important to make this determination before we attempt to introduce an integral approach where it may not fit.

4. The Integral Relationship

The integral relationship is the foundation of an integral healing practice. It is vastly different from the customary practitioner- and diagnosis-centered relationship. Consider the conventional practitioner-patient relationship depicted in Figure F.

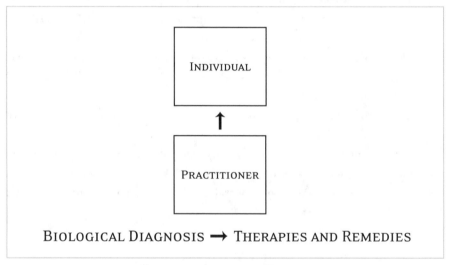

Figure F. The Conventional Practitioner-Patient Relationship

Here the practitioner elicits information from the patient that is relevant to his or her approach. An Ayurvedic practitioner would elicit different information than a Chiropractic practitioner or a conventional Western practitioner. In most instances, the information elicited is usually shaped by the perspectives of the practitioner and limited by our cultural preoccupation with the physical and biological. The aim is to gather the proper information, make a diagnosis within the particular practitioner's system, and initiate the corresponding therapy. The practitioner and his or her approach determine the character and scope of the interview.

Now consider the integral relationship depicted in Figure G.

Here the practitioner and the patient are joined in a healing partnership. Information isn't elicited in the customary manner of question and response. The practitioner and patient sit together in deep listening as the individual relates his or her

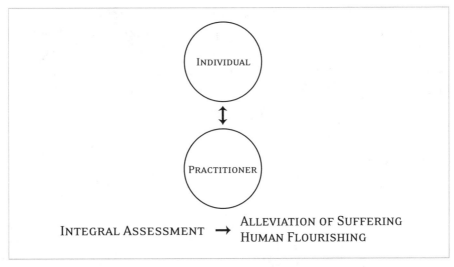

Figure G. The Integral Practitioner-Patient Relationship

concerns. The listening continues until the communication has arrived at its natural end. The healer and healee are joined in a healing community whose sole aim is to seek the full truth of this individual's life for the purpose of alleviating suffering at its source and promoting human flourishing.

Deep listening can only occur in the still mind. The active mind is subject to a continuous movement of thoughts, feelings, and images that interpret and bias what is heard. The still mind is free of these mental movements, and therefore it is also free of their contaminating influence. We listen with the totality of our being. There is no separation between the speaker, the listener, and the listening. If your entire being is listening, the listening itself will become meditation. In this way, we experience the truth of this person's life. We experience it in our mind and body. And from this we arrive at a comprehensive and empathic understanding of their presenting concern. This understanding naturally and effortlessly forms itself into a program for change. This truly holistic and evolutionary understanding of the patient allows for an integral approach.

When listening in this way, even more occurs. By filling our still self with the other's experience, we become aligned with our patient's life. We are truly empathic and compassionate. The other can feel this acknowledgment. He or she can sense our presence and the sense of being cared for, held, and acknowledged. Few of us have had even short periods of such complete presence and attention in our lifetime. For a moment, imagine what it is like to be deeply acknowledged in this way. In itself, this is quite healing.

Similar to how the practitioner takes on the patient's experience, the patient takes on the practitioner's stillness. Gradually, the patient experiences a growing inner stillness. By the end of the meeting, both individuals feel the calm and stillness of the subtle mind. This is a marker that deep listening has occurred. At this moment, the practitioner can point out the quality of the still mind, its ease, peace, and clarity. For many, this is the first introduction to contemplative practice.

Here is a list of the characteristics of deep listening:

Characteristics of Deep Listening

1. Sense of intimacy

2. Empathy

3. Compassion

4. Unity of heart and mind

5. Direct knowledge of the other

6. An acknowledging presence

7. Mutual inner peace and stillness

The integral relationship is the way we build trust and communion. It initiates the healing process, provides the knowledge needed to develop an integral "diagnosis and prescription," and introduces the patient to contemplative practice.

5. The Integral Diagnosis

The integral diagnosis emerges from information gleaned from the initial session and any appropriate testing. As you've probably guessed, what we are calling a diagnosis here is quite different from customary use of this term. It is more like arriving at an understanding of the unique essence of the individual's life. We are seeking together to answer the following two questions: What are the causes of suffering in this individual's life? What are the opportunities for human flourishing?

The integral diagnosis falls into two major categories that correspond to the horizontal and vertical aspects of the integral model. First, we consider how each aspect of the individual's life contributes to suffering and can contribute to healing. This is a holistic approach to the presenting concerns. Second, we seek to identify potential areas of future growth and development. In this way, the integral perspective is two-dimensional; it is both truly holistic and evolutionary at the same time. It integrates both.

6. The Integral Prescription

When identifying the aspects of the individual's life that would be the most advantageous to address, we may find that one aspect needs attention because it represents a major source of suffering and another because it offers the most promising area for growth and development. A direction is chosen based on this assessment, and an integral program is developed that addresses all four quadrants of the patient's life.

An integral prescription is a living experience. It must address the outer and inner aspects of our experience, be tailored to the individual, and be open-ended. At times, we may focus more on temporary relief and at other times on permanent relief through developmental practices. The progress of the program requires continuous monitoring, with shifts and fine-tuning as the patient changes. We must always be willing to adapt to changing circumstances even when this may mean a radical change in the program. We must focus on the patient rather than on our tool kit.

7. THE SETTING

Integral practice takes place in three important settings. The integral practitioner must be attuned to each of them. The first is the presence of an open heart, the second is the presence of a clear and unconditioned mind, and the third is a welcoming physical setting. The outer setting is important, but it is meaningless unless the first two inner conditions are met.

The first two are achieved through the practitioner's inner practice. The outer setting is arranged to reflect the openness, warmth, heart, and sacredness central to this process. A welcoming environment helps to set the mind and heart at ease, facilitate intimacy, and convey a feeling of sacredness. Your intention will be communicated to the patient by both your presence and your office setting.

ONE THOUSAND HANDS

When you have clearly chosen this adventure, understood the theory and principles of integral health, and started your personal practice, you are ready to begin an integral practice. The first question may likely be, "How do I do this with such a busy practice? Where do I begin?" As I have suggested earlier, if you are already in a busy practice, set aside time after your regular hours one day a week to listen to a patient's complete story.

With this individual, practice listening from an open and still mind. Allow the process to unfold without concern or anxiety about where it is going. When you are unclear, don't assume or interpret, ask. Focus on the interaction itself, the listening, the acknowledgment, and the communion that is occurring between you. At the conclusion of the interview—and do not set an artificial time limit—engage your patient in planning a multidimensional approach. First, determine what is necessary to temporarily relieve immediate suffering. Then, determine what steps need to be taken to heal suffering at its root source. Finally, consider what steps can assist this individual in moving toward integral health. If you do this once a week, you will learn a great deal, and I am certain that your soul will be deeply nourished.

In the East, the great healer is often depicted with one thousand hands. This signifies the need for every integral healer to have many ways in which to reach out to meet the unique needs of each individual. So we are taught to have a thousand or tens of thousands of ways to help. In this depiction of one thousand hands, each palm is painted with the eye of a wise healer. This is to remind us that determining the proper way to help requires great insight and wisdom. Each circumstance is different and continuously changing. "Will our temporary efforts support or hinder a deeper healing?" "Where are the openings?" "What is a match for the capacities of this individual?" These and many more similar questions will provoke deep thoughtfulness.

It is essential to respect the complexity of health and healing. Humility is a great virtue. We are not yet fully enlightened healers. But we can begin to learn to respond to others with wisdom, skill, and compassion, seeking to relieve suffering and assist with the attainment of sustained health, happiness, and wholeness. We will not master this art quickly. As Hippocrates, the father of Western medicine, said, "The art is long and life is short." But we can begin. And that is what makes all the difference.

THE INTEGRAL VOW

When we start a fitness program or change our diet, we identify the changes we wish to make, we set goals, affirm our intention, and commit ourselves to this change. This serves to inspire, guide, and support our new efforts. When change is raised to the sacred level of caring for ourselves and others we refer to this as a vow, as a sacred vow. So let us take a sacred vow that takes us directly toward integral health and practice.

As an integral practitioner, I commit myself to:

- Enter a personal process of self-development. I recognize that this requires an inward turn that is supported by the necessary changes in my outer life and is grounded in regular contemplative practice.

- Study, understand, and integrate an integral vision and its principles and practices into my personal and professional life.

- To hold a vision of health and healing whose final goal is health, happiness, and wholeness—a possibility that exists for every person regardless of individual circumstances. I recognize that health and healing in this expansive sense can continue up to and through death.

- Uphold the ethical principles of a spiritual life. In general, this can be defined as those attitudes and behaviors that serve to eliminate suffering and promote peace, health, happiness, and wholeness for ourselves and others.

- Meet every individual as a unique sacred being. The individual's circumstance, needs, temperament, and capacities will define the personalized process of health and healing. I recognize that deep, unconditioned listening is necessary to achieve this goal.

- Develop through personal contemplative practice a healing presence that is acknowledging, comforting, reassuring, safe, nonjudgmental, and infused with loving-kindness.

- Acknowledge and support the innate healing capacities in each individual. I recognize that the individual is the ultimate source of his or her health and healing and the author of his or her own life.

- Hold all life as unique and precious.

- Serve.

May you be blessed
in your life and work.

Resource Guide

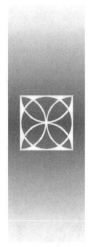

I want to provide you with a list of resources that will deepen the experience we have begun together in this book. Because the integral approach is person-centered, that puts certain limitations on recommending particular resources. I would prefer to sit down with each of you to hear your needs and to find a proper fit. That is how it should be done. But we cannot do that here so I will try my best to describe each of these resources. That will allow you to decide if it is right for you. I will also limit my recommendations, giving you the responsibility to explore further resources. Do not hesitate to try a book, a workshop, or another experience, but if it doesn't fit, just let it go. That's how it should be.

I am listing these resources in the order I suggest you consider them.

CONTEMPLATIVE PRACTICES

A CD of the major practices in this book can be obtained through Dr. Dacher's website: www.elliottdacher.org.

BOOKS

Integral Theory

Wilber, Ken. *Theory of Everything.* Boston, Massachusetts: Shambhala, 2000.
This is a concise and comprehensive overview of Ken Wilber's integral theory. It is essential reading for those who wish to delve deeper into this work.

Psychospiritual Flourishing

Wallace, Alan. *Genuine Happiness*. Hoboken, New Jersey: John Wiley and Sons, 2005.
The author provides a clear and practical introduction to contemplative practice. The reader will find in Genuine Happiness a more detailed explanation of the practices we have discussed and presented in this book.

Salzberg, Sharon. *Loving-Kindness: The Revolutionary Art of Happiness*. Boston: Shambhala, 1997.
This important book fully covers the practices related to the ripening of a personal and universal loving-kindness. It is an essential book for our work.

Muller, Wayne. *Sabbath*. New York: Bantam Books, 1999.
This lovely book is a heartfelt inquiry into the place of silence and solitude in daily life. Exercises are included in the text. I highly recommend it.

Goleman, Daniel. *Destructive Emotions*. New York: Bantam Books, 2003.
This book is an account of a meeting that took place in 2000 with the Dalai Lama, Western scientists, and contemplative scholars. It is an opportunity to sit in on a rich conversation about consciousness, contemplative practices, and health.

Seligman, Martin. *Authentic Happiness*. New York: Free Press, 2002.
As you may recall, we emphasized that psychological health was a foundation for spiritual development. Dr. Seligman takes us through the emerging field of positive psychology, articulating the elements of a healthy psychology.

Biological Flourishing

Murphy, Michael. *The Future of the Body*. New York: Jeremy P. Tarcher/Putnam, 1992.
In this book Michael Murphy provides an extensive study of the evolution of human capacities. He offers a bridge between the psychospiritual and biological aspects of life. The scope of its inquiry and the length of the book make it appropriate for those who want to dive more deeply into the origins and extent of human capacities.

Interpersonal Flourishing

Levine, Stephen and Ondrea, *Embracing the Beloved*, New York: Doubleday, 1995.
Using as a background their relationship and work with other couples, Stephen and Ondrea Levine have articulated the path to spiritual intimacy. Here a "cave for two" substitutes for a "cave for one." The relationship becomes the spiritual teacher. I am unaware of any other book that covers this possibility as thoroughly and passionately.

Wilber, Ken. *Grace and Grit*. Boston & London: Shambhala, 1993.
Ken and Treya Wilber share with us a remarkable and touching account of the psychospiritual development of their relationship during Treya's five-year struggle with cancer. With honesty and clarity, we are given a window into the profound possibilities of intimacy and spiritual union.

Flourishing in the World

Whyte, David. *The Heart Aroused*. New York: Doubleday, 1994.
Using corporate America as a teaching laboratory, the author speaks to the place of soul and spirit in the workplace. He urges and shows us with poetry, myth, and a deep heart how to find creativity, passion, and meaning at work.

Parker, Palmer. *The Courage to Teach: Exploring the Inner Landscape of a Teacher's Life.* San Francisco: Jossey-Bass Publishers, 1998.
Here we could easily substitute the word "healer" for teacher. This book is a touching and well-considered guide to returning heart and soul to the healing process—a book not only for teachers and healers but for all of us who wish to infuse our work with meaning and purpose.

For Practitioners

Carlson, Richard, et al. *Healers on Healing.* New York: Jeremy P. Tarcher/Putnam, 1989.
Prominent healers were asked by the author to identify the golden thread that runs through the healing process. The result is this fine book. Their answers form the chapters: Love, Wholeness, The Healer Within, The Healing Relationship, Consciousness and Healing. It is a wonderful discussion of the core of healing.

Needleman, Jacob. *The Way of the Physician.* London: Penguin, 1982.
The book is currently out of print, but it is worth a library visit. The author, a noted scholar and philosopher, weaves a compelling story that takes us back to the past and into the future in the search for a more profound understanding of health and healing. He speaks from the practitioner's perspective.

Schlitz, Marilyn, Tina Amorok, and Marc Micozzi. *Consciousness and Healing: Integral Approaches to Mind-Body Medicine.* St. Louis, Missouri: Elsevier-Churchhill Livingstone, 2005.
This text covers many issues related to consciousness and health, including several articles that offer a variety of perspectives on integral health.

Ryan, M., and Edward Deci. *On Happiness and Human Potential: A Review of Research on Hedonic and Eudaimonic Well-Being.* Annual Review of Psychology. In S. Fiske (ed.), *Annual Review of Psychology,* Vol. 52 (pp. 141–166). Palo Alto, CA: Annual Reviews, Inc.
This is an excellent review article on eudaimonic theory, the theory of human flourishing. You can download it from the auther's web site.

RETREAT CENTERS

A useful way to explore contemplative practice is to begin with a week or a weekend retreat. There are many options. I have included two recommendations that I know you can count on for care, knowledge, and skill.

The Insight Meditation Society
1230 Pleasant Street
Barre, Massachusetts 01005
Phone: (978) 355-4378
Email: www.dharma.org

The Spirit Rock Meditation Center
P.O. Box 169
Woodacre, California 94973
Email: www.spiritrock.org

The Shambhala Centers
www.Shambhala.org
I have a particular fondness for the Shambhala centers. First, they can be found in almost every major city in the world. Second, they offer a well-designed, well-taught, and largely secular introduction to human flourishing and contemplative practice. This program is offered over a year in 5 weekend trainings. It can be extended the second year to an advanced 7 weekend trainings. You also have the option of attending topical programs. Most important, you will find a supportive community of like-minded individuals.

RELATED ORGANIZATIONS

Integral Institute
integralinstitute.org
This site, developed by Ken Wilber, has a large range of resources related to integral theory and its applications.

Institute of Noetic Sciences
101 San Antonio Road
Petaluma, California 94952
(707) 775-350
www.noetic.org
Good resource for information on consciousness-related conferences, research, and education.

Mind and Life Institute
www.mindandlife.org
Good resource for information on the interface of contemplative practice and Western science.

Gross National Happiness Project of Bhutan
www.bhutanstudies.org.bt/

Genuine Progress Index for Atlantic Canada
www.gpiatlantic.org

These two sites will introduce you to a Western and an Eastern effort to promote the flourishing of an entire culture. The premise is that health, happiness, and wholeness are the final aims of life and thus should be the central concern of society. Browse these sites and read the thought-provoking and uplifting papers.

Acknowledgments

We live in a world of interconnected experience. It would be impossible to acknowledge the endless threads of experience and contributions from individuals that have helped shape this book. It is clearly not my effort alone. I am merely a conduit for understandings that far exceed my own. I will mention here the individuals that have most directly inspired and supported the writing of this book.

I've previously referred to my two medical educations. I would first like to honor those women and men who have taught me the magnificent science of Western medicine. Two come to mind. Both are in the lineage of internal medicine, which has been my specialty. The first is Sir William Osler, whose instructions came to me through his writings. The second is Bernard Lown, whose teachings came to me during my residency years at Harvard. What they taught me was that science and humanism are the inseparable ingredients in the formation of a master healer.

I would also like to honor the people of Tibet and their brilliant and giving wise ones. They have developed and cultivated an extraordinary understanding of the heart and mind, which has been joyfully and sincerely shared in mentorship and friendship. I wish to express my endless appreciation to His Holiness the Dali Lama for the many teachings I attended at his monastery in Dharamasala. Geshe Rinchen Sonam, Geshe Dawa, and Ruth Sonam were the wonderful teachers at the Tibetan Library of Works and Archives. Others whose formal and informal teachings have contributed to this second medical education are Tosknyi Rinpoche, Tai Situpa, and Tenzin Palmo.

I would like to thank Ken Wilber for his many years of creative work in developing and articulating integral theory, which has been the backbone of this book. It would be difficult to separate my interest in integral theory from the inspiring and brilliant writings of Sri Aurobindo.

For many years the Institute of Noetic Sciences has been at the forefront in the exploration of consciousness and healing. I appreciate their presence and support. More recently I have been enriched by the ongoing work of the Mind and Life Institute in its exploration of the interface of Western science and Eastern contemplative practice.

Jeanne Fredericks has been my steadfast agent for many years, and I am ever thankful for her patience and support. Susan Davis edited this manuscript. Her devotion and care has made this book far more user-friendly. Norman Goldfind at Basic Health Publications was sufficiently perceptive and willing to move toward the future of healing. I admire and appreciate his foresight.

A special thanks is due to Elaine Adams, Harriet Cianci, and Mike Zych for their efforts in producing the audio CD of the contemplative practices in this book.

Most important are those friends who have supported me with their love and care—Terese Reamer, Peggy and Marty Albert, Simona Bodo, Katia Cedar, Alok and Gita Chopra, Tami Dawson, Steve Horowitz, Jay Hughes, Rita Marsh, Heather Rynd, Brenda Sanchez, Barbara Stewart, Teena Dhyan Summers, and Eva and Stephen Weinstein.

Final thanks go to my two amazing children, Alison and Jessica, and Harvey Stoller and my late sister, Kay Stoller.

Index

Aging, 127
Aloneness, 55–56
Art. *See* Creative art and expression.
Asclepius, 11, 26, 56
Assessment, integral, 105–116, 151
    principles of , 105–106
Awareness, 22, 39–41, 141

Behavior, control of, 52–54
Bhutan, 46
Biofeedback, 81, 83
Biographs, 112
Breathing, 66, 68–69, 75, 81, 98
Broadhead, W. Eugene, 87–88

Calmness, 40, 54–56, 65–66, 73
Campbell, Joseph, 127
Cause-and-effect, 134–135
Center for Human Flourishing, 147–154
Childhood, 140
Cognition, 107
Compassion, 22
Consciousness, 7, 9, 13, 15–23, 30–31,
    38, 39–41, 46–47, 59–62, 71–78,
    93–94, 119, 130–131, 140
    calm-abiding, 40, 61, 65–66, 73, 75,
    76, 98–99

sensorimotor, 39–40, 61
unity, 40–41, 61–62, 74, 75, 76–77
witnessing, 40, 61, 73, 75
Contemplative practice. *See* Practice,
    contemplative.
Cortex, 20–21, 22
Creative art and expression, 45, 103,
    125

Death, 10, 43, 86, 127
Disease, 127
    heart, 37, 84
Dynamism, 124

Eliot, T. S., 62, 155
Emotions, 19–20, 63, 108
Epidaurus, 27–28

Focal points, 75, 76, 92
Focus, 75–76, 115
Frankl, Viktor E., 100–101
Fry, Christopher, 157
Fulfillment, 45

Gamma waves, 63
Generativity. *See* Teachers and teaching.
Genuine Happiness (Wallace), 78

Gibran, Kahlil, 102–103
Grace, 128
Grey, Alex, 84, 125
Gross National Happiness, 46
Gurus, 121

Happiness, 46, 141–142, 144
Healers. *See* Practitioners.
Healing, 11, 12–13, 15, 23, 26–32, 48,
    94, 98, 101, 120, 129–135, 150,
    166–173
  Aesclepian, 26–32, 152
  See also Health, integral;
    Practitioners.
Health
  biological, 132, 143, 159–160
  integral, 9, 12–14, 18, 25–32,
    35–48, 118, 129–135, 142–144,
    145, 147–154, 151, 156–157,
    166–173
  ordinary, 130, 131, 132
  See also Medicine.
Heart disease, 37, 84
Heraclitus, 134
Human development and experience, 7,
    8–9, 12, 14, 105–116, 131,
    139–146, 155–157
  biological, 41–43, 80–84, 108, 132
  dynamic, 47–48, 106, 124, 133–134
  evolutionary, 37–46, 74, 129, 133
  holistic, 36–37, 79–86, 114, 129,
    133, 140–141
  intentional, 38, 46–47, 101, 129, 133
  interpersonal, 43–44, 51–52, 87–94,
    108–110
  people-centered, 47, 98, 99, 133
  psychospiritual, 39–41, 59–69,
    84–86, 106, 107–108, 112,
    140–141
  worldly, 44–46, 53–54, 55, 95–103,
    110–111, 129

Human flourishing, 129, 131–132,
    139–146, 147–154

Individuals and individuality, 47–48,
    119, 133
Integral Practice Program, 12, 122–124
Intimacy, 90–92, 126

Jung, C. G., 60

Learning, Greek, 26–29
Life-as-practice, 121, 124–127, 152
Listening, 106, 150–151, 168–170
Lotus flowers, 78
Loving-kindness, 50, 51–52, 65, 66–69,
    93, 98, 101, 119, 134, 142

Magritte, René, 125
Man's Search for Meaning (Frankl),
    100–101
Martial arts, 83
Medicine, 159–164
  Buddha, 11–12
  holistic, 162–163
Meditation. *See* Practice, contemplative.
Mental imagery and visualization, 17,
    144–145
Mental training, 16–23, 63–64, 65–66,
    68–69, 79–84
Mind/body, 12–13, 15–23, 42, 63,
    79–86, 130
Motivation, 107
Munch, Edvard, 125

Nature, 125
Negativity, 53
Neuropeptides, 17
Noise, 54–56
Nutrition, 108

One thousand hands, 171–172

Oneness, 89, 93–94, 126, 135, 169–170

Pain, 83
Physical fitness, 81, 82, 108
Potential, 37–38
Practice
    contemplative, 50, 54–55, 62–69, 72, 82–83, 119, 122, 124, 134, 141, 142, 151
    integral, 66–69, 75–78, 92, 94, 124–128, 132, 134, 144–145, 151–152, 153–154
    preparations for, 66–68, 78
    principles of, 118–121
    subtle mind, 71–78
Practitioners, 123, 150, 152, 167
Prophet, The (Gibran), 102, 103
Psychoneuroimmunology (PNI), 16

Qigong, 81, 83

Relationships
    dependent, 90
    integral, 168–170
    interpersonal, 43–46, 51–52, 87–94, 126–127, 142
Relaxation, 81, 83
Renunciation, 55–56
Retreats, 66, 68, 149–152
Reverse entrainment, 151, 170
Rilke, Rainier Maria, 89, 102
Rothko, Mark, 125

Sacred Mirrors, The (paintings), 84–85
Sanctuaries, 150

Self, 56–58, 64, 74, 86
Self-centeredness, 51, 52, 69, 91
Separateness, 93
Service, 45–46, 95–96, 97, 99
Sexualitiy, 126
Silence and stillness, 54–56, 68–69, 71–72, 73, 76, 82, 92, 169
Spiritual body. See Spirituality and spiritual body.
Spiritual union, 90–93
Spirituality and spiritual body, 25, 40–41, 42–44, 61, 84–86, 101, 132
Sri Aurobindo, 158
Stress, 18–19, 20–21, 84, 87, 96
Subtle mind practice. See Practice, subtle mind.
Suffering, 134

Tai chi, 81, 83
Teachers and teaching, 110–111, 120, 126, 129, 130, 132
Three pot metaphor, 167–168
Transformation, 100, 101–102, 124–125

Virtue, 119
Visualization. See Mental imagery and visualization.

Wallace, Alan, 78
White, John, 85
Wholeness, 140–141, 144–145
Wilber, Ken, 35, 112, 166
Work, 95–103

Yoga, 81, 83

About the Author

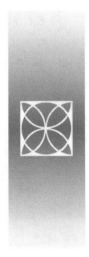

Photographer: Onkar Singh Jaryal

Dr. Elliott S. Dacher received his medical degree in 1970 and practiced full-time internal medicine for twenty-one years. He is the author of *Whole Healing* (Dutton, 1996) and *Intentional Healing* (Marlowe, 1996). He is a past fellow of the Institute of Noetic Sciences and has served on the editorial board of the *Journal of Complementary and Alternative Medicine*. Currently, Dr. Dacher studies, practices, and teaches the principles and practices of integral health and healing. He continues to counsel individuals aspiring to use distress, disease, and life itself as a pathway to an integral health.

Born in New York City in 1944, Dr. Dacher now lives in Massachusetts. He has two daughters, Alison and Jessica.

You can contact Dr. Dacher at esd@elliottdacher.org, or visit his website at www.elliottdacher.org.